MILLI
MENOPAUSE

MILLENNIAL MENOPAUSE

Preparing for PERIMENOPAUSE, MENOPAUSE & LIFE'S NEXT PERIOD

LIFE'S NEXT PERIOD

LIFE'S NEXT PERIOD

LIFE'S NEXT PERIOD

LAUREN A. TETENBAUM
LCSW, JD, PMH-C

ULYSSES PRESS

Text copyright © 2025 Lauren A. Tetenbaum. Design and concept copyright © 2025 Ulysses Press and its licensors. All rights reserved. Any unauthorized duplication in whole or in part or dissemination of this edition by any means (including but not limited to photocopying, electronic devices, digital versions, and the internet) will be prosecuted to the fullest extent of the law.

Published by:
ULYSSES PRESS
an imprint of The Stable Book Group
32 Court Street, Suite 2109
Brooklyn, NY 11201
www.ulyssespress.com

ISBN: 978-1-64604-810-6
Library of Congress Control Number: 2025930777

Printed in the United States
10 9 8 7 6 5 4 3 2 1

Acquisitions editor: Claire Sielaff
Managing editor: Claire Chun
Copy editor: Renee Rutledge
Proofreader: Paula Dragosh
Front cover design: Akangksha Sarmah
Interior design: Winnie Liu
Layout: Abbey Gregory

NOTE TO READERS: This book has been written and published strictly for informational and educational purposes only. It is not intended to serve as medical advice or to be any form of medical treatment. You should always consult your physician before altering or changing any aspect of your medical treatment and/or undertaking a diet and/or exercise regimen, including the guidelines as described in this book. Do not stop or change any prescription medications without the guidance and advice of your physician. Any use of the information in this book is made on the reader's good judgment after consulting with their physician and is the reader's sole responsibility. This book is not intended to diagnose or treat any medical condition and is not a substitute for a physician.

To my grandmother, Ilene Abrams Tetenbaum.

You helped inspire my appreciation for women's stories and the passion for writing my own.

CONTENTS

- INTRODUCTION: **WHY MENOPAUSE, WHY ME?** 1
- GLOSSARY: **SOME LINGO** 12
- CHAPTER 1: **PERIOD, START OF STORY** 16
- CHAPTER 2: **MILLENNIALS, MEET MENOPAUSE** 26
- CHAPTER 3: **OUR MOTHERS' MENOPAUSE** 48
- CHAPTER 4: **MENOPAUSE IN THE MEDIA** 68
- CHAPTER 5: **FROM PREGNANCY TO PERIMENOPAUSE** 83
- CHAPTER 6: **YOUR BODY, YOUR CHOICE(S): MENOPAUSE AND MEDICINE** 95
- CHAPTER 7: **WOMEN'S HEALTHCARE IN AMERICAN CULTURE** 137
- CHAPTER 8: **MENOPAUSE AND MENTAL HEALTH** 152

CHAPTER 9: BEAUTY, BODY, BRAINS—AND PERIMENOPAUSE 178

CHAPTER 10: LET'S TALK ABOUT SEX 205

CHAPTER 11: PERIMENOPAUSE AT WORK 216

CHAPTER 12: MILLENNIAL MEN AND MENOPAUSE 231

CHAPTER 13: GIRL POWER 244

CHAPTER 14: WHAT'S NEXT AFTER WHAT'S NEXT? 254

CHAPTER 15: MILLEN*OPAUSE* 275

CONCLUSION: HOW CAN MILLENNIALS PREPARE FOR MENOPAUSE? 286

RESOURCES AND ADDITIONAL READING 294

ENDNOTES 297

ACKNOWLEDGMENTS 330

ABOUT THE AUTHOR 334

Introduction

WHY MENOPAUSE, WHY ME?

Get in, millennials, we're going through menopause.

Menopause is coming. Millennial menopause, millenopause, millennialpause, Generation Y's menopause—however you want to label it, and whether you knew it or not, it is upon us.

What is millennial menopause? It's a moment, and it's a movement. Millennials are, in general, about to be menopausal, yet most of us have no idea what that involves. To me, "millennial menopause" describes the menopause transition experienced by millennials. Now let's talk about what that actually means.

Members of the millennial generation can be characterized as born between 1981 and 1996[1]—we'll go with that definition plus a few years on either end of the range for this book (but anyone at any age is welcome to read it, especially our xennial sisters who are a few years ahead!). Women usually go through menopause between the ages of 46 and 55.[2] So, if you identify as a millennial and you're reading this in 2025 or later, you are likely in your 30s or early to mid-40s and may have recently realized you should be thinking about menopause.

You may be years away from your final menstrual period—but the menopause transition, I have learned and want you to know, can start long before then. By 2030, the number of menopausal and postmenopausal women in the world will be around 1.2 billion.[3] These days, given that the average life expectancy for females is about 80 years,[4] most women in the United States live approximately a third of their lives postmenopause.

If you're a millennial like I am, you may be minimally knowledgeable about menopause. Yet menopause is inevitable for all those who have experienced puberty and gotten their period, and who are fortunate enough to reach a certain age.

But what determines that age? When do symptoms of menopause start, what exactly are they, and how long do they last? How do we know if we have entered into the menopause transition? How do we treat menopause symptoms? What happens after menopause? Why isn't menopause talked about more in mainstream media, by healthcare providers to women in their 30s and 40s, and among women themselves? What can we do to prepare for menopause?

I admit: Until recently, I wasn't sure. Honestly, I had no idea. I didn't even think to get prepared, despite my typical overachieving tendencies that I (used to) proudly refer to as "type A+." Not too long ago, it occurred to me that I knew way too little about what was going to happen next to my body, my health, my mood, and my life.

Shortly before my 39th birthday, I got invited to attend a professional women's networking event in my hometown of New York City, sponsored by the nonprofit UJA-Federation of New York. The evening's topic was "The Trailblazers of FemTech," and panelists included reproductive health start-up founders. I chose to attend a breakout session led by Anne Fulenwider, the cofounder and co-CEO of Alloy, a digital health company changing the menopause conversation, because I like to learn and felt like I had a lot to learn about menopause.

Within minutes, I recognized that "a lot to learn" was quite the understatement.

As Fulenwider shared her story about how her mother's sudden death sparked her passion for women's health advocacy, I realized I knew next to nothing about menopause. And I am a clinical social worker specializing in women's mental health during their reproductive years. I am highly educated and fairly well-read. I am fortunate to have great doctors. I'm not shy about talking about women's bodies. When I was in college, I taught sex education to middle school students and interned at Planned Parenthood's corporate office, where I contributed to marketing campaigns to raise awareness about reproductive health. So why did I know so little? And if I knew so little, what about my peers? My clients? I was astonished by my own ignorance in that moment, but the women around me reassured me it wasn't my fault.

In that menopause informational session, I was the youngest participant by at least a decade, if not two, on average. There were other millennials at the larger networking event, but it seemed like they didn't yet recognize the significance of this particular topic or its relevance to our age group. But I was glad to be able to learn from my elders. I was struck by the way they passionately agreed with Fulenwider about how they had gone years feeling unheard and ignored, even by top healthcare providers in their fields. I noticed their resentment toward the media for spreading misinformation about menopause treatments. I heard their pleas for more information to be shared, for more access to options.

I cheered internally when Fulenwider described with confidence: "Millennials won't be dismissed. This next generation is comfortable being loud to get what they need and deserve. As they approach menopause, they will demand accessible, high-quality treatment and accurate information. They will speak up."

But then, I thought: *Who will speak up for us? I haven't yet heard anything at all about menopause. Who will be our voice, the voice we so desperately need, as we approach the next chapter of our lives and our health?*

And later, I realized: *Me. I can and I will be part of that voice.*

I didn't expect to be some kind of magical menopause messenger as I approached midlife, but I felt motivated to learn more. And I wanted to share what I learned. Science is not a strength of mine, but using my voice—my words—to advocate for women's rights, equality, and empowerment certainly is.

ME, A MAJOR MILLENNIAL

I am proudly a millennial. I was born in 1985. I grew up with Mary-Kate and Ashley. When I was a child, the adults around me wore puffy sleeves and even puffier hair. We listened to Raffi's children's music on cassette tapes and later watched Barney on TV. In elementary school I devoured books from *The Babysitter's Club* and *Sweet Valley High* series. I remember when the Soviet Union collapsed and exactly where I was when OJ Simpson got arrested and later acquitted. As an adolescent I knew (and still know) every episode of *The Fresh Prince of Bel Air* and *Saved by the Bell* and related to nearly all of the main female characters on the WB's/CW's lineup (Buffy, Felicity, Joey—you're my girls). The biggest love triangles of my time have included Jacob and Edward, Aidan and Big.

I got an AOL account at age 12, using it to log in via dial-up modem and argue with my brother, two years my junior, over how much time we could each spend taking a turn on our family's shared computer. Back then, having your own phone landline and personalized answering machine was the coolest. As a young teen, I was obsessed with the Spice Girls and boy bands (I'm your girl for any *NSYNC trivia contest). I didn't fear Y2K and the supposed computer crash that was coming for us, but I did recognize the specialness of living during the turn of a century.

My later high school memories are marked by September 11 and the invasion of Iraq—and my first phone, a Nokia device with a thick plastic case that I changed depending on which colors were available at the mall. Texting was barely a thing but the snake game was all that and a bag of chips, as we used to say (cringe). I was among the first of my generation to get a Facebook account in college, a time when we considered our technology highly advanced if our (non-flat-screen) TVs had VCRs *and* DVD players. My sister, a millennial who was born in 1990, used social media to discuss homework assignments on classmates' walls (are they still called that?). We all posted dumb photos to digital albums, thinking a camera phone was rare and sophisticated—remember "Muploads"?

When my generation entered the workforce, it was during the great recession, a time when we used BBM pins to communicate and online dating was brand new (as in, one had to type in "www." on an actual computer), not quite yet universally available via apps and certainly not yet the norm it has become. Because of the technology we created and demanded, industries like journalism and advertising have been transformed; for better or worse, the world is now used to more personalized marketing and instant gratification. Millennials have been criticized for being lazy and entitled at work, but we were the ones who made ourselves accessible to work all the time via smartphones and WiFi and a cultural attitude shift. Many of us millennials were parenting young children when COVID-19 hit, forced to figure out homeschooling and isolation as we were struggling to build our careers, all while knowing we may not do as well financially as our parents did because the economy, and the world, had changed.

As Fulenwider had alluded to, we millennials were comfortable (more than generations prior, at least) talking about how hard it all was—maybe because it was actually harder for us or maybe simply because we had learned that in order to create change, we needed to speak up.

Millennials have been loud about fertility and mental health struggles. We have contributed to if not led the advocacy related to ending the gender pay gap, promoting women in politics and STEM, speaking out against sexual harassment, and accessing better, more tailored healthcare. We've created more comprehensive personal care product and service offerings, and we've helped destigmatize LGBTQ+ relationships. We're still working on all these, but we're working hard.

And yet, as my 30s were coming to an end and I felt ready to embrace whatever was coming in the next decade, no millennial I knew was talking about menopause. Maybe it's because it seemed early, sure, but I learned about periods and sex and giving birth well before I actually experienced any of those transitional life moments. I read about puberty and sexuality in the *What's Happening to My Body?* book—complemented, of course, by Judy Blume's fictional masterpieces like *Are You There God? It's Me, Margaret*, *Forever*, and *Summer Sisters*. I read about pregnancy, parenting, and partners in caregiving in books like *What to Expect When You're Expecting*, *Good Inside*, and *Fair Play*—books that provided answers to my questions any time of day (or night), books that made me laugh when I was near (or in) tears, books that made me feel seen and heard. These were books I shared with other women, our sticky notes creating rainbows as if we were studying for an exam, though we knew there was never just one right answer.

But where was the book about menopause for millennials, my generation?

Well, girlfriends, here it is.

WHAT TO EXPECT WHEN WE'RE EXPECTING MENOPAUSE (OR WHEN WE DON'T EVEN KNOW TO EXPECT IT)

This book is meant to be a sort of menopause manual for millennials. It's meant not only to educate you on what you may feel and what to do about it, but also to teach you why our generation has been taught so little about menopause and how we can make change. If you were embarrassed to pick up a book with "menopause" in the title, all the more reason for you to read it—and share it. We shouldn't be shamed for wanting to learn more about our next phase of life, whether it has already started for us or will in several years. We should take pride in being proactive.

This is a book in which I've collected and interpreted the most current information (as of 2025) and connected with the foremost professionals in women's health to give you—and myself—real and relatable insight into what our generation can expect regarding what's next. As a therapist and advocate, I have counseled hundreds of women (mostly millennials) experiencing shifts in mood, values, and perspectives. The ways our reproductive health—and our reproductive rights—impact women's autonomy, identities, and opportunities are immeasurable. And reproductive health includes menopause.

So this is a book that will help millennials prepare for menopause to the extent that we can, to go into this new chapter equipped with information, resources, and optimistic and curious attitudes. This is a book full of the ideas and experiences of dozens of women, women who did not hesitate to share because they wanted to help other women.

The great author and Nobel Prize for Literature winner Toni Morrison said back in the '80s (perhaps the best decade ever, according to many millennials), "If there's a book that you want to read, but it hasn't been written yet, then you must write it." I ended up writing the book I needed. I hope you find it helpful, too.

I want to emphasize the first and most frequently proclaimed piece of information I was provided in my numerous conversations with countless women, including a variety of women's health experts: *"Menopause is experienced differently by each and every woman."*

Each woman will have her own experience with symptoms, with their severity and impact or lack thereof, with various health factors and risks and goals that may affect her decisions around treatment options, and with how she chooses to approach this period of life.

Accordingly, this is not a book that will tell you what to do when it comes to your personal menopause journey. This is not a textbook full of medical jargon, but it will show you where to look if you want that. This is not a book that will address every possible medical risk or symptom. This is not a book written by a physician or medical professional.

But this is a book written by someone who has dedicated her personal and professional life to supporting women. This is a book written by someone who cares deeply about women's health (including mental health), quality of life, and ability to make choices for themselves. This is a book that will illuminate topics that have previously been in the shadows and that will provide resources and data to point you in the right direction so you can learn more as needed or desired. This is a book that you can rely on for basic information about what you didn't even know you should know. This is a book through which I wish to inform and encourage you, to inspire you to speak up for yourself and your changing needs as you navigate the menopause transition.

My hope is that this is a book that will be there for you like a trusted friend, with all the support Blair and Serena gave each other (without any of the bullshit). This is a book that will help guide you through a major life transition that can be lonely and scary, but does not need to be.

As a social worker specializing in life transitions affecting millennial and young women—and a millennial mom myself—I know intimately how important it is to feel you're not alone when you're experiencing a hardship or even a seemingly minor life adjustment of some kind. I can't count the number of times I've heard, "It's so helpful to hear other women experience this, too." Whether it's in connection with dating or partnerships, family dynamics, career stressors, family planning ambivalence, postpartum loneliness, breastfeeding frustration, body image issues, or mental health and mood disorders—it is incredibly reassuring to recognize that you are not experiencing a monumental life shift in isolation.

Menopause—like adolescence or even womanhood in general—is a unique experience, but it is a universal one. We may all go through it at different times and in different ways, but I can say with certainty that we should be talking about it. We should be learning from each other. We should be preparing for it together.

As I underwent my own journey to learn more about my next life stage, I felt compelled to write this book because I know the strength of sharing. I know the magnitude of women imparting wisdom, the comfort of going through a big change with a community of support. And like I said, I'm not shy about this stuff. (For context: As an undergrad, I shouted, "Vaginas are here!" on the University of Pennsylvania's main campus pathway, Locust Walk, to promote my participation in the play *The Vagina Monologues*; while in law school, my nickname was "Condom Girl" because I ran a fundraiser selling condoms and candy for charity as president of the Law Students for Reproductive Justice club.)

My mission is and always has been to support and empower other women. I believe it is time we do that when it comes to menopause.

So, will you talk about it with me? Will you learn with me? Will you get ready with me for what's next?

I hope so.

Let's go, girlies.

Glossary

SOME LINGO

Here's how I define some terms and labels I use frequently throughout the book.

AARP: An interest group in the US focusing on issues affecting people 50+ years old (formerly known as the American Association of Retired Persons).

ACOG: American College of Obstetricians and Gynecologists, a professional organization of physicians specializing in obstetrics and gynecology.

Birth Control Pill ("The Pill"): A hormonal oral contraceptive used to prevent pregnancy and regulate menstrual cycles.

CBT: Cognitive behavioral therapy, a form of psychotherapy in which unhelpful ways of thinking and/or behaving are modified to more effectively manage stress and other symptoms of depression and anxiety disorders.

CVD: Cardiovascular disease, the term for a group of disorders affecting the heart and blood vessels; CVD is the leading cause of death among women in the United States.

FDA: Food and Drug Administration, a federal agency of the US government's Department of Health and Human Services, dedicated to protecting public health by regulating items like medications.

FemTech: Products and services that use technology to address women's health issues.

FMP: Final menstrual period, a year after which a woman officially reaches menopause.

Genitourinary Symptoms: Those that affect the urinary and genital organs (including vulva, vagina, and bladder), often referred to by the umbrella term "genitourinary syndrome of menopause" (GSM).

HRT: Hormone replacement therapy, the former common term for menopausal hormone therapy (MHT), which is now preferred and more accurate (since hormone therapy does *not* typically *replace* hormones to be back to premenopause levels).

HT: Hormone therapy, an abbreviation for menopausal hormone therapy.

IUD: Intrauterine device inserted into a woman's uterus to prevent pregnancy.

Menopause Transition: The life stage marked by changes to a woman's menstrual cycle or other peri/menopause symptoms, culminating in menopause.

Menopause: The date a woman reaches a full calendar year without having a period.

The Menopause Society: Formerly the North American Menopause Society (NAMS), this organization's mission is to empower healthcare professionals "to improve the health of women during the menopause transition and beyond."

MHT: Menopausal hormone therapy, i.e., hormonal treatment that can come in various dosages and forms, including oral medications and transdermal patches, to alleviate symptoms. As mentioned, this is now the preferred term by clinicians over "hormone replacement therapy," or "HRT," unless hormone levels are actually being replaced (e.g., due to early menopause). Throughout this book, I'll use "MHT" and "hormone therapy" or "HT" interchangeably (and use "HRT" when referred to as such by the original source).

Millennial: A person born around 1981–1996.

Perimenopause: A diagnosis describing the time around menopause, characterized by fluctuating hormones and a variety of potential emotional and physical symptoms; this phase can last for several years.

POI: Primary ovarian insufficiency, a condition in which a woman's ovaries stop functioning normally before the age of 40.

Postmenopause: The time period after a woman reaches menopause; i.e., the rest of her life.

UTI: Urinary tract infection, a common and painful bacterial infection occurring in the urinary tract.

Vasomotor Symptoms: Symptoms like hot flashes or night sweats caused by hormonal changes disrupting a woman's body temperature regulation.

WHI: Women's Health Initiative, a series of clinical studies, including the 2002 study on hormone therapy (Chapter 3 will discuss how this study has since been followed up on and clarified).

Woman: A person with female reproductive organs who has menstruated; this book has been written with the awareness and understanding that not every person who identifies as a woman has had a period nor does every person who has had a period identify as a woman, and the conviction that *all* people deserve compassionate care.

Chapter 1

PERIOD, START OF STORY

• • • • • • • • • • • • • • •

Do you talk about your period with your girlfriends? How about with your sexual partners? With your kids? Do you ever talk about it with the men in your life who are not family? What about those who are?

Menstruation is a natural part of life. In fact, it could be considered the source of life. One cannot get pregnant without being able to ovulate, a phase of the menstrual cycle in which an egg is released from an ovary. Getting her period for the first time is a pivotal moment in any girl's adolescence. It's as old as time, yet still often shrouded in secrecy, shame, and even disgust.

I noticed as much when my family's puppy got her period. It was quite a coincidence, actually. I had recently told my kids, then aged eight and five, that I was writing a book about menopause. I explained it as a moment in a grown-up woman's life when her body changes and she can no longer become pregnant because she stops getting her period.

"OK but … What's a period?" they asked, entirely unfamiliar despite our household's fairly open dialogue about bodies. They didn't know much because I hadn't gotten mine in nearly six years, due to the hormonal IUD (intrauterine device) I'd had inserted in my uterus soon after my daughter was born. I had only recently decided to remove the contraceptive device to have a sort of bodily reset, and had yet to menstruate. (Note: Not everyone skips bleeds altogether while wearing a contraceptive device, but it is quite common for women with hormonal IUDs to have very light or nonexistent periods.)

"A period is something that girls get when their bodies go through puberty, usually when they're preteens or young teenagers," I explained. "It means she's able to get pregnant and have babies one day. A period is blood that comes out of a girl's vagina." My then-kindergartner daughter looked scared. "It doesn't hurt though, it's not like a scrape or a cut," I clarified. "It's just part of her body. She can wear special underwear or use special things called pads or tampons to help stop the blood from going everywhere. It's all very normal."

Within 24 hours of this conversation with my children, our dog began to bleed. "She got her period!" I told my kids excitedly, marveling at the opportunity to show them in real life what we had just been discussing in the abstract. I also thought it was really funny and cute to see the dog in her little diaper. Together as a family we put our pup in special diapers accompanied by menstrual pads I had stored, untouched, in a closet for years. I joked with my mom that since the dog had become a woman, I wondered if I was supposed to lightly slap her across the face like she had done to me, an old Jewish tradition.

And then, only a couple of days later, I got my own period for the first time since early 2018, which felt like a lifetime ago. I told my kids and they took it in stride. We went to the pharmacy to get more feminine products for both me and the dog. We openly and unabashedly talked about it all.

"Can the dog walk with us to school today?" asked my son. "I think I'll keep her home because she has her period," I replied, not intending to go into the nuanced implications of a dog in heat strolling through the neighborhood while we got through our morning routine. "But you're able to walk and do regular things and you have your period," he rightfully observed.

When my daughter had a friend over to play, she advised, "The puppy is wearing a special diaper right now. It's because she's bleeding, because she has her period. My mommy has her period, too. Don't worry, it doesn't hurt them. It's not scary or embarrassing. It's just part of their bodies."

I swelled with pride (and maybe a bit of bloating). I felt proud that we had such open and direct conversations about menstruation—about science and facts—in our family. A couple of years earlier, I had been quoted in *The New York Times* for having a similar nonchalant approach to biological basics.[5] Back then (which my son had since forgotten by the time our dog menstruated because periods were not part of our daily life), I explained that the main character in the Disney animated film *Turning Red* "got her period 'because that's what happens to girls when they become teenagers.'" My son's response? "OK, cool."

But in 2024, I realized not everyone shared my direct approach or attitude of acceptance. When I told a friend born in 1987 that our dog had gotten her period, she asked, "Was your husband like, 'Ewww, what is this?!'" No, he was not. He knew what a period was, and he shared my approach to openly communicating with our kids about reproductive health. He also readily changed the puppy's pads and period diapers as part of caring for her. This friend has three young daughters. I hope she doesn't expect her husband to react in shock and dismay when they get their periods—and I doubt he will—but time will tell.

Another friend, who was born in 1980, reacted to the animal anecdote with a simple yet exclamatory text: "Gross!!!!!" *Was it really?* I wondered. I admit, it's not exactly fun to deal with cleaning up any bodily fluid, but as parents—and humans—we've all dealt with our fair share, because well, that's just how bodies behave. I later inquired about how this friend was handling conversations with her middle school–aged daughter about periods. She said, "I've spoken about it with her, and emphasized she can come to me with any questions she has, especially if she hears things from her friends or from school that might be confusing." I responded, "Nice. What about coming to her dad with questions?" My friend replied, seemingly stumped, "Well, sure, she could do that. I just hadn't thought about it."

When my millennial peers and I got our periods, it felt like something to hide from the rest of the world, even though among ourselves we anticipated and embraced it as a rite of passage. In public, we literally *would* hide tampons and panty liners up our shirtsleeves while going to change them in the school bathrooms because it was unheard of to simply hold the items in our hands. We'd slip our gym teachers notes from the nurse excusing us from swim class, blushing as they read them, nodded, and discreetly allowed us to sit on the sidelines (though looking back, the reason must have been obvious). "Check the back of my pants," we'd whisper to each other as we stood up while on our cycle. Having a leak in which one bled through her bottoms in public was the most agonizing thing we could imagine.

By the time we were in high school, for me, it all felt a little less secretive. I always had many male friends with whom I felt close enough to complain about painful cramps or feeling grumpy. I'd say nearly all of the guys very much knew what was involved during "that time of the month when we surfed the crimson wave," as pop culture referenced. And thankfully it wasn't just the boys with sisters who had an open mind. My first serious boyfriend had only a little brother, yet, out of respect for me and my body, he never blinked at my keeping tampons in the bathroom at his parents' home.

However, the progress my generation has made regarding the rhetoric around menstruation pales in comparison to the centuries of shame and stigma women have endured. Even some of the oldest religious texts imply that menstruating women are "unclean" or "impure." Women and girls are still too often treated differently—treated poorly—for having their periods. It used to (and still does) make me sad on their behalf when my friends revealed that their partners refused to have sex with them while on their periods because they felt it was "nasty." Of course, if a woman isn't in the mood or just doesn't want to because of her period or otherwise, she shouldn't. But I firmly believe she shouldn't be made to feel like she is disgusting and undesirable for simply experiencing her menstrual cycle, simply existing as a female human with bodily functions.

And a female with bodily functions who is aging experiences even more stigma. In popular culture, she's regarded as a foolish old woman when having a hot flash, if she's paid attention to at all. In real life, she's often met with awkwardness and aversion if she tries to raise awareness about what she's enduring. Yes, much of menstruation as a topic is personal, but it is still a commonly shared part of human development. If we overlook the conversation about that journey, we can (and do) easily ignore what comes after. As it stands, we're still not talking enough about menopause.

HOW CAN MILLENNIALS PREPARE?

Talk About Women's Health

There are consequences to the hush-hush nature of the way we discuss menstruation and the shame that we project onto young women—actually, women of all ages—who are experiencing it. There are impacts on women's mental health, self-esteem, and bodily autonomy. Every woman I know who has experienced painful periods, hurtful sex, an abortion, infertility, a miscarriage, pregnancy, labor, parenting, or any reproductive health issue always says this upon sharing: "It feels much less lonely to talk about it." As a culture, millennial women and men alike have become more open about their experiences, more accustomed to sharing their private struggles in the hopes that they can help others and get answers for themselves.

We have to keep (or start) talking about menopause, and about our health in general.

It can start with talking about periods. In a 2023 study, more than three-quarters (76 percent) of teens reported the desire for more open communication about their periods and admitted to being curious or confused about their menstrual cycle.[6] When we have visible, comprehensive conversations about these issues, we help normalize them and improve access to needed care.

We may be moving in the right direction in some public forums, which helps normalize the topic in more private ones. In July 2024, ahead of the Summer Olympic Games, the underwear brand Knix (whose motto for its teen line is #BleedConfidence) took out a full-page ad in *The New York Times* as part of its campaign, offering to pay athletes to talk about their periods in order to destigmatize having one. In September 2024, Katy Perry performed a medley of her greatest hits at MTV's VMAs* before accepting a lifetime** achievement award and announcing she was doing it all on the first

---

* BTW, let's take a moment to honor the beautifully simple afternoons of TRL music video countdowns.
** Katy! You're one of us. You still have so much lifetime left!

day of her period. Love to see it! I hope that we can continue to get more comfortable talking about extremely natural physiological processes, including menstruation and menopause.

When I started my research for this book, I asked 120 friends, acquaintances, and anonymous survey participants to consider their experience of talking about menopause. Fellow millennials born in 1985 noted, "It's not talked about at all," and, "It feels like it's taboo." A 1979-born mom I know emphasized, "Menopause is like a huge mystery. But it doesn't have to be." A friend born in 1972 who experienced early menopause shared, "Menopause is a subject that needs to be discussed in more detail at a younger age."

Indeed. As Joan Rivers used to say, "Can we talk?"

Normalize Menstruation (and Its End)

I acknowledge that every family, household, or setting has different practices around conversations connected to bodies, bathroom activities, and anything related to sex or reproductive health. I am not here to insist there is one way to have these conversations. I may never be able to convince you that it shouldn't be awkward for a preteen to discuss her period with her father. You may never have a husband who unhesitatingly picks out period products for you at the drugstore.

But I do hope I can help you rid yourself of the shame of having a body that menstruates, and that one day will no longer. I hope that the women in my generation—and our daughters in the next—will no longer feel humiliated by their periods (or lack thereof).

A woman born in 1976 told me that she wants "to encourage women of all ages to share their experiences of their pregnancies, hormones, periods, perimenopause, infertility, and postpartum, to help support each other's feelings." I agree. When we openly share information, we help normalize very normal experiences. We remove stigma and build self-confidence. We empower each other and ourselves.

As with periods, menopause, conceptually, holds extra layers of shame. It's not just a woman's issue that isn't prioritized, or a bodily issue that creates embarrassment, but also a reflection of age. And let's be honest, we are uncomfortable with aging in our culture, especially for women. It's nearly impossible to go online or watch TV without seeing some type of ad promising to stave off the effects of aging in some way, as if we are doing something wrong by daring to continue to live and grow. A friend born in 1981 reflected, "Society makes menopause sound like a full stop. Birthdays should make us feel powerful and important, but instead women get cast aside as they age. Why? This ageist outlook is killing women's confidence." She's right.

While menopause does signal the end of fertility and certain bodily functions, it should not be a source of disgrace. You may not want to shout about your menopause, but I encourage you to talk about it the same way you might a physical ailment like a headache (which maybe you've had luck treating with certain medication or wellness practices), or a psychological transition like moving to a new town (it can be hard and lonely but also interesting and an opportunity to reflect). Talk with and learn from your friends. You might find online communities like forums or private groups on social media helpful. Share resources and dispel misinformation. Be open about menopause.

Remember, as my young daughter indicated: It's not scary or embarrassing. It's just part of your body.

Chapter 2

MILLENNIALS, MEET MENOPAUSE

After I attended the event with Anne Fulenwider, I went to my friends feeling simultaneously inspired and ignorant. "What do you know about menopause?" I inquired, wondering if I had missed the memo. Did I somehow block out a chapter from 9th grade biology? (I'm a woman of words, not science, after all.) Had I been too distracted by pregnancy and postpartum and career building to think about what was coming next for my body and health?

Turns out I was not the only one. "I know nothing," was the general response among at least 20 millennial friends. One friend said, "That I'll be in a bad mood for a decade," while another answered, "That we're doomed."

Yikes. Was it really going to be that bad, or was the fact that it was life's next big unknown making it more daunting? And even if it wasn't imminent (though, who knew if it was?), shouldn't we have *some* kind of idea of what to expect?

I set out to learn more. I interviewed experts like Arielle Bayer (a board-certified OB/GYN and reproductive endocrinologist and fertility specialist at CCRM Fertility New York), Alicia Robbins (a board-certified OB/GYN, certified menopause practitioner, and founder of The Elm, a boutique women's health practice for women in New York and Connecticut), and Brenda Green (a nurse practitioner and the cofounder of Follaine Health, a New York City–based practice offering personalized treatment to perimenopausal and menopausal women). I gathered my thoughts and their advice and wrote an article, "Are You There Menopause? It's Me, a Millennial Mom," for online platform Mama Beasts' March 2024 e-magazine issue.[7]

Following the article's publication, I received dozens more questions and words of encouragement. "I didn't even know I had to think about this! Thank you for raising it," said one friend born in 1982. "Are we actually old enough for this?!" asked another, who was born in 1984.

Yes, I think we are old enough, or at least, old enough to start getting prepared. I then surveyed 120 peers to assess gaps in knowledge. "What do you want to know about menopause?" I asked. The responses consistently reflected the need for information, any and all information. "I don't even know what to ask. That's how little I know about it!" reflected a woman born in 1989. "I have all the questions, every question," noted a woman born in 1979. Another born in 1986 summed it up simply with: "I truly don't know anything."

And the lack of information was infuriating. I found a 2019 study revealing that over 80 percent of women under 40 either have "no knowledge at all" or just "some knowledge" of menopause; women (particularly those over 30) are angry, even "furious," and frustrated about their lack of education, feeling that "menopause education is essential because it is a 'key part of half the population's lives.'"[8] A woman born in 1982 expressed to me: "I'm so frustrated there isn't much accessible, accurate information about this before we go through it." A friend born in 1985 said, "I really wish we were talking about this more, earlier. It's shocking how little we know about something that can impact us so much—and of course, is a natural part of a woman's life. It shouldn't be that hard to talk about."

Friends, I am with you. I didn't know much either. I had a lot of questions, and the women around me had a lot of questions. So I set out to get our questions answered. Thankfully, the four dozen experts I subsequently spoke with to get these answered meant it when they said, "No judgment."

Based on knowledge I gained from countless conversations with experts and everyday women, resources from The Menopause Society and other professional organizations, information from multiple scientific journals, numerous advanced professional trainings I've taken, various news articles, and guidance from Dr. Bayer, who has been my friend since before puberty, let alone perimenopause, please allow me to present my version of Menopause for Millennials 101. Here are our questions, answered.

MENOPAUSE FOR MILLENNIALS 101

Remind me about the basics of a woman's body parts?

When Bailey yelled about her "vajayjay" in season two of *Grey's Anatomy*, I cringed a bit while watching from my college dorm room, and not because the character looked like she was in pain while giving birth. It was because it felt like yet another cutesy and inaccurate word was being imposed upon us instead of simple, straightforward (and accurate!) terms for female sex organs. And this was before the "vajazzling" craze (I always love an opportunity for extra sparkle, but that was definitely an interesting trend).

Language matters, and I think we have to get comfortable with using proper terminology so that we can get less uncomfortable talking about women's sexuality and reproductive health in general. So, let's clarify—in as simple terms as possible—what we're going to be talking about here.

The vagina is the tube-like muscular organ that can stretch to accommodate a wide range of things going in (like a tampon or penis or finger) and things coming out (like menstrual blood or a baby). The vaginal opening is just one part of the vulva, which is the accurate term for the external female genitalia that include the clitoris (stimulating this sensitive area leads to pleasure, so get to know it!), the hymen, the labia majora and minora (or "vaginal lips"), and the urethra opening. Women have three openings in their genital area: the vagina, the urethra from which they pee, and the anus from which they defecate.

The vagina ends at the cervix, an internal organ that opens (or "dilates") during vaginal childbirth and is the entrance to the uterus. The uterus is a muscular, pear-shaped organ whose inner lining is shed monthly (i.e., during one's period). Often called the "womb," the uterus is also the place where a fetus is held and grows during pregnancy. Inside a woman's pelvis, her uterus is surrounded by (typically) two ovaries, which are glands that contain all of one's eggs ("ova") and the primary female reproductive hormones, estrogen and progesterone.

How does the female reproductive system (including the menstrual cycle) work?

Those two reproductive hormones can be considered the stars of the menstrual cycle show. Among other bodily influences, progesterone helps regulate menstruation, build bone and muscles, and support pregnancy. Estrogen also helps regulate the menstrual cycle and has numerous other benefits for the body, including on the cardiovascular and neurological functions and the skeletal system.[9]

There are three major forms of estrogen, including estradiol (E2), which is the primary form during a woman's reproductive years, during which the ovaries are the primary source of estrogen. The adrenal glands on top of the kidneys and fat tissues throughout the body also secrete estrogen. There are estrogen receptors all throughout a woman's body (as well as in a man's body)—not just in the uterus and breast tissue, but also in the brain, bones, and cardiovascular and nervous systems. This is why the estrogen withdrawal during the menopause transition can affects us throughout our bodies. "Basically," Dr. Bayer explained to me, "when estrogen travels through the body it connects with the receptor cells on all different organs to make different parts of the body work in different ways."

The ovaries are also a main source of progesterone, which also gets secreted from fat (adipose) tissue in a woman's body. There are also secondary female hormones that help regulate the menstrual cycle. The main ones are luteinizing hormone (LH) and follicle-stimulating hormone (FSH), which are both secreted by the pituitary gland in the brain. Women also produce testosterone in the ovaries, adrenal glands, and fat tissue—but in much lower amounts than men do.

During puberty, female hormones change (estrogen, LH, and FSH levels rise), and girls develop breasts, grow pubic hair, and get taller, among other bodily changes. Females become able to reproduce once they get their period (begin menses). The term "menarche" describes a girl's first period, which per my memory, typically occurred between ages 11 and 14 for most millennials. These days, girls in the United States are getting their period earlier on average, a trend that has been shown to be more pronounced in girls of color and from lower incomes, due to a variety of potential factors often dubbed "hormone disruptors," including stress, increased rates of obesity, processed foods, or pollutants that can disrupt the endocrine (AKA hormonal) system.[10]

The average menstrual cycle is about 28 days long, counted from the first day of bleeding. The first 14 days are known as the follicular phase, during which FSH and LH travel from the brain to the ovaries, stimulating the emergence of eggs (in "follicles" similar to shells) in the ovaries. Typically, only one follicle will emerge as the "dominant" or biggest one during this time. ("Think of it as the 'chosen one' for that month," suggested Dr. Bayer.) The rest of the follicles that are not used will disintegrate, and those eggs will be lost.

Females are born with all the eggs they will ever have, so egg quantity diminishes from the time of birth until menopause, when it ultimately reaches zero. During the follicular phase, when the dominant egg is emerging, estrogen levels are also rising. At about 14 days, when the "chosen" egg is ready (or mature), estrogen is at its peak, LH surges, and ovulation occurs, causing a follicle to release its egg from the ovary. "When the follicle ruptures open, a small amount of fluid can sit at the bottom of the pelvis, and some women feel this ovulation pain very sensitively, while others may never notice it," observed Dr. Bayer. Then the egg finds its way to the uterus via the nearest fallopian tube.

If the egg meets sperm in the fallopian tube, it can be fertilized and begin to divide into more and more cells, now called an embryo. "This developing embryo should continue to travel from the fallopian tube to the uterus over the next five days, and if it finds a comfortable place to settle and implant in the lining of the uterus, a pregnancy can begin," Dr. Bayer described. The emptied-out follicle shell in the ovary is called the "corpus luteum" and will continue to support this ongoing pregnancy by producing estrogen and progesterone during the next phase of a woman's cycle, known as the "luteal phase."

If the egg is not fertilized, the egg goes on down the uterus. Along with blood, tissue, and other secretions from the uterus, the egg will ultimately exit through the cervix and vagina. "Put simply," summarized Dr. Bayer, "the woman gets her period."

What does my period do for me?

Your period may bring with it stained underwear, bad moods, headaches, body aches, acne, hunger, cravings for certain foods, irritability, exhaustion, cramps near your abdomen, and other physical and emotional symptoms in the week leading up to and/or of menstruation. But despite Aunt Flo's BS, we tend to appreciate the old gal, because your period reflects fertility, i.e., the capability to get pregnant and reproduce.

I've heard the period described as a conversation between a woman's brain and reproductive organs, or as a monthly check-in with the rest of her body. When a woman gets ill or has undergone a physical change (even if she simply flew on an airplane), her period can be affected and her menstrual cycle can look different than it usually does. When I meet with new therapy clients, or if long-standing clients are experiencing new symptoms, I always ask for information on their menstrual cycle. It can tell us a lot about what's going on for women physically, emotionally, and otherwise, especially if the menstrual cycle has undergone recent changes.

OK, so what if I do begin to notice changes to my menstrual cycle?

Track your cycle so that you become aware of any changes. As aforementioned, an average cycle is 28 days, but that may not (or ever) be true for you. Note what is your "regular" to the extent possible plus any shifts to it.

Changes to your cycle can be due to temporary factors like travel or medication. If you've been experiencing amenorrhea (the absence of menstrual periods) for a few months and you are not pregnant, you should check in with your healthcare provider. If your doctor rules out other causes to cycle changes, you may be in perimenopause.

Peri who? What is perimenopause?

The prefix "peri-" means "around" or "about"—accordingly, perimenopause is the period of time around "natural" or "spontaneous" menopause (meaning, occurring on its own vs. being induced due to surgical procedures or medical treatments[*]). Perimenopause covers the time leading up to and including one year after a woman's final menstrual period (FMP). You may think of perimenopause as the pregame to menopause—a pregame during which a lot more may happen compared with the main event.

Perimenopause typically involves various physical and emotional signs like menstrual irregularities, hot flashes, and mood swings. The changes to your menstrual cycle during perimenopause can include longer or shorter cycles or lighter or heavier flow. Usually in early perimenopause, periods (that are not regulated by hormones in the form of birth control) become irregular by seven or more days. In later perimenopause, toward the FMP, you'll usually skip months of having your period, and cycle lengths can be 60 or more days. But there is no one defining symptom or menstrual cycle pattern that indicates or signifies perimenopause. We will learn throughout this book that the menopause transition is different for each and every woman!

---

[*] I don't like indicating that induced menopause is "unnatural"—similar to how I believe medicated labor is not "unnatural"—so I personally prefer the term spontaneous.

I like the way The Menopause Society defines perimenopause: "Perimenopause is the mirror image of adolescence, which is the coming on to the reproductive years, whereas perimenopause is the coming off of the reproductive years."[11]

There are lots of reasons you may not have heard the term "perimenopause" until recently (or until right now). It may be at least partly because, due to a variety of factors we'll review, healthcare providers generally have been trained to treat women postmenopause, and not in the phase prior to the FMP. Accordingly, it often feels like no one knows WTF is going on with our bodies at this life stage. A 2024 survey of more than 700 women aged 35 to 52 throughout the United States revealed that the majority (60.8 percent) weren't sure whether they were in perimenopause, even though one in four reported perimenopause symptoms beginning before age 35.[12] Perhaps you relate.

Neither perimenopause nor menopause is a disease or a disorder. Rather, the terms can be used as diagnoses of symptoms that reflect the changes your body is undergoing, symptoms from which you may need—and deserve—relief.

What's the difference between perimenopause and menopause?

When we colloquially use language like "menopausal" or "in menopause," we are often actually referring to perimenopause. As aforementioned, perimenopause is the life stage leading up to and including that year post-FMP. The majority of this book will focus on perimenopause, though we will also explore what happens after.

Perimenopause is a clinical diagnosis referring to a phase of life that can last many years. During this time, a woman's reproductive hormones fluctuate. Specifically, in early perimenopause, estrogen is volatile while progesterone declines; periods are usually closer together. In later perimenopause as a woman approaches her FMP, estrogen levels decline. Periods are spaced out and women tend to experience symptoms like hot flashes and vaginal dryness.

Menopause, in contrast, is *one day* that takes place 12 months after your actual last period, or FMP. You won't know that it was your final menstrual period until the full 12 months have gone by without bleeding again (and if there are no other medical causes to this change in your cycle). So, menopause is a retroactive diagnosis.

When a woman reaches menopause, her fertility is officially finished. Per Dr. Bayer, "Her ovaries stop releasing eggs, the production of estrogen and progesterone in the ovaries declines, and she is no longer able to conceive." Once a woman is postmenopause, she is always postmenopausal.

When does perimenopause start?

I'm going to give you an (annoying, sorry) answer from my previous career as a lawyer: It depends.

The most consistent thing I've learned about perimenopause is that it is inconsistent from woman to woman. The symptoms, the age at which they begin, their intensity, and the length of time they last are extremely varied. And because perimenopause is a transitional phase, it's not like it starts at one moment; rather, it is a span of time marked by a variety of symptoms, which women experience at a variety of levels. Some women do not suffer from symptoms at all!

Because of the variability of the perimenopause phase, we don't have an exact number for its duration. It is often said that perimenopause usually lasts for four to eight years. However, most of the providers I spoke with agree that perimenopause begins about eight to 10 years before the final menstrual period (so usually, on average, in a woman's 40s). Menopause specialists are now encouraging medical providers to initiate conversations about anticipating the menopause transition with all women aged 35 to 40 or older so that they feel more prepared for perimenopause, which is likely more impending than previously recognized.[13] It's probably not that women are experiencing perimenopause for longer than what has been captured in the medical literature, but rather that women are (thankfully) increasingly aware of—and comfortable with seeking help for—how they're feeling.

So when should I expect menopause to happen?

Everybody (literally, every body) is different, but as of 2024, the average age of menopause in the United States is 51 according to most experts and women's health organizations. "The age your mother experienced menopause is the best predictor of when you'll go through it," explained Dr. Bayer.

Note that when we talk about menopause, we often talk about women's health at midlife, which is generally the period of life between 40 and 65 and the time at which she'll experience menopause symptoms. I know it can feel weird to acknowledge we are at or approaching middle age, but, here we are.

Other than changes to my menstrual cycle, what are some signs that I've started perimenopause?

While some women may experience very few symptoms during perimenopause, others may endure a wide range that can affect their physical and mental health. "Studies show that about 85 percent of women experience some menopause symptoms," shared Dr. Bayer. And your symptoms can vary day to day and can change as you approach menopause.

Common physical indicators of perimenopause include "vasomotor symptoms" like hot flashes, which the majority (experts usually say 80 percent) of women transitioning through menopause experience. A hot flash can feel like a sudden rush of heat to the face and chest, usually lasting up to five minutes. I've heard hot flashes can feel like a sudden urge to vomit while profusely sweating. One woman told me it feels like "fire traveling down your body, out through your extremities." Another described it as having a cloud of thick heat over her body. I know this is not the *That's hot* energy Paris was always talking about, but I want to be honest.

Other common symptoms during perimenopause can include a variety of sleep problems,[14] including difficulty falling and/or staying asleep, insomnia, or night sweats, which are hot flashes that occur while you're sleeping and can result in wet clothes that make you wonder if you've peed on yourself. Women often report waking up in the middle of the night, perhaps multiple times, and not being able to go back to sleep. There are so many other issues during midlife that may impact sleep, including psychosocial factors and stressors, that can create a cycle of poor sleep and potentially more severe perimenopause symptoms. As I'll discuss, poor sleep can affect nearly all physical and mental functioning.

Other physical symptoms of perimenopause may include vaginal and urinary tract changes (leading to painful sex due to vaginal dryness and/or increased risk of urinary tract infections, or "UTIs"), acne, achy muscle or joints, brittle nails, low back pain, dry or itchy eyes, and weight gain despite no changes in diet or exercise. Additional symptoms can include mood swings, feelings of impatience and rage, anxiety or depression, and fatigue. Experts usually say approximately 60 percent of women report memory problems or concentration struggles, often described as "brain fog," in which women struggle to recall words or anecdotes or names or whether they turned off their (very millennial) flat iron; they describe feeling confused or like their brain is being hijacked.[15]

If I don't get my period, how will I know when I'm in perimenopause?

There are a number of reasons why a woman may not bleed during her menstrual cycle but still not have reached menopause. She may have a hormonal IUD that leads to no regular bleeding, or perhaps she is on the birth control pill and is unaware of her natural, unregulated cycle (or skips a bleed altogether).

Sometimes, due to certain cancers, risks, or conditions like endometriosis (where uterine lining-like tissue grows outside the uterus, typically causing pain and sometimes infertility), a woman will get a hysterectomy in which her uterus is removed. Following the removal of the uterus, she is no longer fertile (as she now lacks a womb), and she will no longer menstruate, but she still has ovaries unless she also undergoes an oophorectomy, a surgical procedure to remove one or both of them.*

To determine whether you're in perimenopause, whether or not you experience changes to your menstrual cycle, pay attention to your health in general. Ask your providers questions about any changes and what they may indicate, and whether lab tests might be helpful. (Note: They aren't always necessary, and there is not one test to confirm or diagnose perimenopause.) I encourage you to look for a provider who is well-versed in menopause; you can find one by visiting The Menopause Society's list of certified menopause practitioners.

What is premature or early menopause and why might it happen?

The Menopause Society defines early menopause as menopause that occurs between the ages of 40 and 45 years.[16] This occurs naturally in 3 to 5 percent of the population. Meanwhile, premature menopause

---

* If you didn't quite know what a hysterectomy involves, you are among many women and even medical providers who frequently misuse terms like "total hysterectomy" (removal of the uterus and the cervix), "partial hysterectomy" (removal of only the uterus—not the cervix), or "radical hysterectomy" (removal of the uterus, cervix, surrounding tissue, and sometimes the upper part of the vagina). The procedure removing ovaries is called an "oophorectomy." Learn more: Rachel E. Gross, "You Had a Hysterectomy. What Did the Doctor Leave Behind?" *The New York Times*, last updated December 6, 2024, https://www.nytimes.com/2024/12/02/health/hysterectomy-ovaries-women.html.

is defined as menopause that occurs before age 40; this occurs in approximately 3 percent of women in the United States.

You may be aware of a condition called primary ovarian insufficiency (POI), also a term that refers to menopause occurring before age 40. It used to be known as "premature ovarian failure" but the term "POI" is now preferred (as the term "failure" has negative connotations) and more accurate (since ovarian function could resume). According to The Menopause Society, up to 10 percent of women with POI can get pregnant following intermittent ovulation—so it's not that they are actually in menopause, but rather experiencing POI. POI is a clinical condition affecting approximately 1 to 3 percent of women.

Given the above stats, it's likely that at least a few of the women you know have experienced premature or early menopause. And they are probably feeling confused and lonely, since we so often (incorrectly) associate "menopause" with elderly women. They are also likely at risk of additional health issues, since the ensuing loss of estrogen can put them at risk of heart disease, stroke, dementia, and osteoporosis. So if you find yourself thinking, "Menopause is so far away for my generation," consider this.

And consider if you could be one of those women with these conditions. If you are younger than 40 and experience no periods or many skipped periods, and there is no other medical explanation for it, speak with your healthcare provider about whether this is a sign of POI or premature menopause. The causes of POI or premature or early menopause are not always known. The conditions may be due to genetic disorders including certain mutations; autoimmune disorders like rheumatoid arthritis, HIV, or other infections; or a history of smoking cigarettes. Some believe that extreme stress can trigger early menopause.[17]

Premature or early menopause can also be medically or surgically induced. Essentially, if both your ovaries stop working for some reason, you will enter menopause. One reason behind ovarian dysfunction could be the surgical removal of both ovaries (a procedure called a "bilateral oophorectomy"), which some women pursue to treat endometriosis or prevent certain cancers for which they are at risk. Ovaries may also stop functioning because of medications used to suppress the ovaries and production of estrogen (this can be temporary) or harsher, more permanent treatments like chemotherapy or radiation, which are toxic to the fragile ovaries.

As you can see, the menopause experience is nuanced. It's difficult to give general explanations that would apply to all women. However, I will say this, to all women: Even if you are experiencing menopause earlier than average or earlier than when you might have expected to, you do not have to suffer through your symptoms.

Tell me more … What *can* I do about my symptoms? What are the range of treatments available? When do I need treatment because my symptoms aren't "normal"?

There is no one right way to treat menopause symptoms (the general term I'll use to describe the symptoms you may experience before and after your FMP, including during perimenopause). You should speak with a licensed healthcare provider to try the appropriate treatments depending on your lifestyle, health history, genetics, and other medical needs. And, you should know that a treatment that works in the beginning of perimenopause may not be as effective as you approach your FMP or in the years following due to a variety of reasons (i.e., as your hormones fluctuate, so can your symptoms), so it's important to keep monitoring yourself and maintain an open dialogue with your provider.

In general, treatment options for symptoms in both perimenopause and postmenopause may include prescription drugs like hormone therapies as well as nonmedication options like lifestyle strategies.

Hormones can be prescribed in various forms that will be explored further in Chapter 6, including pills, patches, sprays, gels, injections, tablets, vaginal rings, or creams. Hormones may treat a variety of menopause symptoms, including hot flashes, vaginal dryness, and dips in libido or mood. Menopausal hormone therapy can be extremely effective in treating symptoms but do come with some risks—like all medications do. Women should evaluate their risks, health histories, and symptom management goals with their providers before pursuing hormone treatment.

Nonhormonal therapeutic options for menopause symptoms, which will also be further discussed in Chapter 6 and in subsequent chapters, can include medications like SSRIs (selective serotonin reuptake inhibitors, drugs that increase serotonin levels in the brain), vaginal lubricants, lifestyle habits like not smoking and maintaining a healthy diet, and treatments like cognitive behavioral therapy, which I primarily utilize as a therapist in my practice. Some women use a combination of treatments, or certain treatments for certain periods of time depending on their individual needs.

There is absolutely no one-size-fits-all approach to treating menopause symptoms.

In general, both HT and nonmedication options may help women feel better physically and emotionally—more like themselves before they began experiencing symptoms—and can possibly even help prevent further health problems. But please remember that this is *not* medical advice specific to your situation, so if you want more info, ask your doctor!

As far as knowing *when* to ask for help, I suggest you do so whenever you want or feel you need to or just want to learn more! I won't underestimate how difficult it can be to access a healthcare provider who really listens, and I know that women tend to put themselves last. (*Pediatrician appointment for your kiddo? Done. Annual physical appointment made for yourself? Ehhhh, that's been on the to-do list for a while.*) But when it comes to your health and well-being, you deserve to be your own biggest advocate. There's no threshold you have to cross to receive treatment, no indication of symptoms that are "abnormal" or "too much" that you have to match to get the help you deserve. If and when anything feels different, uncomfortable, or painful, speak up.

Will my race or ethnicity impact my experience with menopause?

Potentially. It's widely known that Black women experience vasomotor symptoms (like hot flashes and night sweats) more frequently and for a longer duration than White or other women. In particular, a 2006 study of more than sixteen thousand diverse women found that Black women reported vasomotor symptoms most frequently, followed by Hispanic, then White, then Chinese, and then Japanese women.[18] But exactly why is still unclear; the results could be due to differences in the way women of various cultures perceive and report symptoms, or, as a 2024 study examined, because discrimination is associated with greater risk of vasomotor symptoms.[19] A different 2024 study of more than sixty-eight thousand women concluded that the severity of symptoms is associated with race and ethnicity, regardless of socioeconomic status.[20]

We must recognize (and advocate to improve) the healthcare disparities affecting women of color in the US. As stated in a 2021 *Journal of Women's Health* article: "The history of Black women's access to health care and treatment by the US medical establishment, particularly in gynecology, contributes to the present-day health disadvantages of Black women. Health inequality among Black women is rooted in slavery."[21] Women of color, including Black women, are too often dismissed or misunderstood when they seek out medical care,[22] and in turn may distrust the traditional medical system in general. So their experience with menopause may indeed be different than that of White women due to biological or environmental or a combination of factors.

And while this book will focus on women in the US, menopause is experienced by women all over the world. The experiences of women in other countries may or may not resemble those in the US. The average age of menopause in India is 47, for example, a bit earlier than in the United States.[23] One woman's experience with the menopause transition will be different from the woman living down the street or across the globe. Yet all women can learn from, teach, and support each other through menopause.

How will my life change after menopause?

I wish I could tell you that after that final menstrual period, you'll return to the energy, health, and optimism of your youth, just without your fertility. Unfortunately, I can't. Symptoms (the ones you experience during perimenopause and/or new ones!) can last for several years after the FMP. Their impact will vary depending on many factors, including how and when you treat them.

After menopause, women may be at increased risk of cardiovascular issues and bone changes, including increased risk of osteoporosis (a disease classified by loss in bone density that causes bones to be more likely to break), diabetes, and certain cancers. Of course, risks for other health issues increase with age, too, so it can be hard to distinguish what is due to menopause or simply due to age. Then again, since menopause is totally natural and has always happened to women, it can be thought of as just part of (instead of distinct from) the aging process.

The good news is, knowing you've experienced menopause and your last period can bring some relief. You can toss your tampons, enjoy sex without risking pregnancy, and appreciate the passage of time without needing to track your monthly visitor. Just like puberty and perimenopause, postmenopause is a natural phase of life.

HOW CAN MILLENNIALS PREPARE?

Build Knowledge

First, congratulate yourself—you've completed Menopause for Millennials 101! Donna Martin graduates and so do you. Oh, the places you'll go!

In all seriousness, I believe the best way to prepare yourself for anything is to build your basic knowledge around it, with the understanding that experiences can be varied—and that's OK. I hope this overview has been helpful for you. If you walk away with only a couple of conclusions, I hope they are that you deserve help if you need it and that knowledge is power.

In the chapters ahead, we'll get more information on how we might be able to prevent or alleviate symptoms and engage in strategies to make the menopause transition as smooth as possible. We'll also work to understand (and dismantle) the secrecy that tends to surround menopause and women's health in general. And, we'll learn why and how we have to advocate for more when it comes to menopause.

For now… Class dismissed! Feel free to play Vitamin C's "Graduation (Friends Forever)" song you got really sick of in high school and now feel nostalgic for. No judgment.

Chapter 3

OUR MOTHERS' MENOPAUSE

Not one of the 120 women I surveyed said they learned an adequate amount of information about menopause from their mothers. Most did not learn anything at all from them. A few can recall witnessing what they now recognize as symptoms, like crankiness and hot flashes. One woman born in 1986 said she could remember her mom was always holding a glass of cold water to her neck but otherwise identified as feeling totally clueless about menopause. Another born in 1980 shared: "It was never spoken about in my household. I just know my mom had really bad hot flashes for a long time." This woman went through menopause herself "very suddenly," yet, "I knew almost nothing … I was not prepared."

Why didn't our mothers talk about their menopause experiences with us? They all went through it, and some clearly suffered from it. And, generally, our mothers had taught us about puberty and pregnancy. So where were our moms when it came to menopause?

Did you talk about menopause with your mom while she was experiencing it? "Absolutely not," answered Kara Alaimo, a millennial mother of two, communications professor at Fairleigh Dickinson University, and the author of the book *Over the Influence: Why Social Media Is Toxic for Women and Girls—And How We Can Take It Back*. "But I don't blame my mother. I think the inattention to it and secrecy around it are part of a much bigger cultural problem."

The bigger cultural problem was (and still is) that women are expected to endure pain and not create a fuss. Our moms were conditioned to believe that their symptoms were just part of growing older, that nothing could be done about them, and that getting older itself was something to feel ashamed and quiet about. "For my mom's generation, the messaging was that 'Your body is no longer doing what it is supposed to do,'" reflected Kara Cruz, a millennial therapist based in California who focuses on marriage and family therapy and perinatal and perimenopausal mental health. "They were made to feel like something was wrong with them if they felt moody or couldn't lose weight they had gained in midlife. They weren't told that it was something happening *to* them, or that they should talk about menopause with healthcare providers so they could access support and resources."

Seeking treatment for mental health or other struggles was perhaps hard enough. Our mothers' own mothers were often overprescribed sedatives in the 1960s and '70s, suppressing their emotions during motherhood and menopause and perpetuating the idea that a woman should be amenable to whatever challenge life threw her way. It's perhaps understandable that our moms didn't really have the words to articulate the challenges they may have been experiencing during their menopause transitions.

Alaimo added, "Our lack of knowledge—or even basic awareness—of menopause care all goes back to this idea in our society that women are supposed to be the ones providing the care, and not cared for. The expectation is that women care for others and not themselves." She referred to a 2009 study that revealed a woman is six times more likely to be "abandoned" (via separation or divorce) soon after a cancer or multiple sclerosis diagnosis than male patients.[24] "I see this trend anecdotally, too," shared Alaimo. "Implicitly or sometimes even explicitly, women are deemed unworthy of being cared for. As a result, women don't want to complain or appear sick or in need. They are effectively silenced."

It didn't help that our mothers were dealing with inconsistent, intimidating, and, it turned out, inaccurate medical information during their menopausal years.

THE 2002 WHI STUDY

In 2002—the year I turned 17 and my mother 46, for context—the Women's Health Initiative (WHI) released a paper about its hormone therapy study (which I'll refer to as the "2002 WHI study") called "Risks and Benefits of Estrogen Plus Progestin* in Healthy Postmenopausal Women: Principal Results from the Women's Health Initiative Randomized Controlled Trial."[25] The trial was one of the largest and most expensive studies funded by the US government's National Institutes of Health.

But the research was halted early because preliminary data suggested that postmenopausal women taking hormones were at increased risk of breast cancer, stroke, pulmonary embolism, and cardiovascular disease. Conclusions were inappropriately drawn about whether hormone therapy in general was safe and effective for women with bothersome symptoms of menopause, which was not the objective of the study—meaning, not what was actually studied. The drugs in the study were synthetic versions of estrogen (specifically, conjugated equine estrogen) and progesterone, effects of which cannot and should not be generalized to all kinds of hormone therapy. Moreover, the trial had major limitations, including that the women studied were mostly over 60, way past menopause (with most participants more than 10 years past their final menstrual period), and already at higher risk of health problems. Individual risk factors like family history were also not properly considered when the faulty conclusions were drawn.

And yet, panic seemed to take over the researchers and anyone who listened to them.

Following the paper's publication highlighting the potential risks (which have since been found to be statistically insignificant), there was a whirlwind of attention from academic and mainstream media.

---

* Progestin is a synthetic version of progesterone.

WHI researchers appeared on televised press conferences and *The Today Show*. Additional media coverage included scary headlines in *CNN*, *The Washington Post*, *BCC*, *Newsweek*, and *The New York Times*. Fear about taking hormone therapy spread among women and their healthcare providers, a legacy that still lingers today.[26] Some medical experts did push back at the time, but their messaging to the public was not communicated widely enough, arguably until very recently. In 2024, the International Menopause Society described the reporting around the WHI study as "a shock to conventional wisdom," since menopausal hormone therapy previously had been viewed positively; further, "the absolute risks of MHT on health outcomes in the WHI were rare to very rare by common standards, [but] the data were alarmingly presented as percentage changes rather than absolute numbers by the media, and the risks were said to apply across all age groups."[27]

Because of the inaccurate messaging, as Adrienne Mandelberger, a millennial and a minimally invasive gynecologic surgeon and certified menopause specialist who founded Balanced Medical, a New York–based gynecology practice, described: "Many women stopped hormone therapy without talking to their doctors, and many doctors stopped prescribing them for fear of backlash or because they were not fully aware of the data." Echoed Caroline K. Messer, a New York–based physician double board certified in internal medicine and endocrinology, diabetes, and metabolism: "Prescriptions for hormone replacement therapy came to a screeching halt." And they are still today not the norm. According to The Menopause Society, as of 2023, hormone therapy use in women aged 40 or older was down to only 1.8 percent [!], despite substantial evidence confirming its safety and potential impact on bothersome symptoms.[28]

As a result of the rhetoric around the 2002 WHI study, "an entire generation of women needlessly suffered," maintained Anne Fulenwider, of the FemTech workshop that sparked my interest in this topic. A 1960-born friend affirmed: "I'm part of the generation that got no information about hormone therapy options because it simply, suddenly became unavailable. I'm part of the generation of women that got screwed."

How terribly sad and unfair for our mothers, who were likely told to stop or were never even offered MHT. How scared and disappointed they must have been when they were advised that nothing could be done to help them feel better. Of course, not all women were impacted by the 2002 WHI study, but it could not have been easy or without distress for the generation that heard the general sentiment that MHT was dangerous.

Today, experts agree that the WHI trial was inadequate on many levels, leaving lasting damage for women, especially for the women who have needed effective treatment for their life-disrupting symptoms.[29] For about two decades, "millions of women were not given basic information about a safe, generically available, affordable option to alleviate their symptoms because the world of hormones had gone dark," lamented Fulenwider. If hormone therapy really were as harmful as indicated following the WHI, we should have seen a great improvement in women's health overall once it stopped being so widely prescribed and used—but we haven't. Instead, the women who may have benefited from hormone therapy have lived in fear and pain because they were unable to access such treatment.

It's not that menopausal hormone therapy must (or can) be taken by every woman, but rather that every woman should understand how and why it might be a treatment option. Every woman should be informed so that she can make her own choices about treatment and quality of life for the rest of her life.

Fulenwider's own mother, Connie, was on hormone replacement therapy but went off it after the 2002 WHI study. Perhaps related to her halting MHT and in turn, its potential cardioprotective benefits (which will be discussed further in Chapter 6), she died suddenly of a heart attack in 2016 at age 73, inspiring Fulenwider to consider how she could make an impact on women's health during the rest of her own life following a successful career in women's magazines. "I was struck by how many women were not given the option," she explained. "No one talked about it, no one was taught it, people were afraid for nearly 20 years."

It wasn't just laypeople who were affected by the study's messaging but also medical professionals and medical policies. Deborah Duke, a lifelong New Yorker and my friend's mom, didn't know any friends who used HRT. "We would have weekly professional education trainings where we'd have speakers and hormone therapy drug reps come," recalled Duke, whose decades-long nursing career in women's health spanned various roles, including as the OB/GYN clinical nurse manager at Flushing Hospital in Queens. "It was the norm to at least discuss hormone therapy as an option for women, and it was often encouraged as a course of treatment. Then in the early 2000s, it felt like the conversations stopped." Following the WHI study, many professionals became skeptical if not scared.

MILLENNIALS NEED MORE THAN OUR MOTHERS GOT

Millennials can learn from what our mothers went through when they were our age. We must continue to advance women's health, though we are today still dealing with a lack of knowledge among healthcare practitioners. As recently as May 2024, menopause expert Dr. Lauren Streicher reiterated the lasting impact of the 2002 WHI study to *PBS*: "Physicians [have] not [been] advising patients to take hormone therapy. They're not comfortable with it. Most physicians, quite frankly, weren't trained in hormone therapy because they trained after the WHI."[30]

Even among the brilliant and exceptionally educated physicians I know, this observation is accurate. More than one provider I tried to interview who attended the very best schools and training programs told me they were embarrassed they could not answer basic questions about menopause treatment. "Women's health felt like an afterthought, and we didn't hear much more than 'Menopause causes hot flashes. Moving on to the next topic …'" one highly trained healthcare professional told me of her purported higher learning.

Another, an OB/GYN who was aware that her own mother had gone through early menopause at 43, shared that she didn't think to identify her night sweats and brain fog as perimenopause symptoms for years while in her late 30s; instead, she suffered through migraines and asked her primary care physician to test her for Lyme disease. After starting a hormone therapy regimen including an estrogen patch and a hormonal IUD, she felt much better physically and mentally almost immediately. Even her hairstylist noticed significant healthy hair growth over the course of just three months. This doctor said she felt foolish for not having connected the dots, but, given her lack of education despite her expertise, it's clearly not her fault.

My friend Dr. Alison Schram, a millennial gynecologic medical oncologist, attended an Ivy League university for medical school and recalls having no training devoted to menopause at all during her studies to become an internist and then a cancer specialist. She told me, "I certainly think this topic deserves more attention from medical schools and professional training programs." In fact, she chose to pursue a career in gynecologic oncology because of the significant unmet need. "Although we have made incredible progress in the treatment of gynecologic cancers over the past decades, advanced gynecologic cancer remains a leading cause of morbidity and mortality for women."

While clinicians like Dr. Schram who focus on women's health give me hope for the future, it's been disappointing to realize how little attention has been paid to our issues thus far. In 2025, it remains an uphill battle for most women to get in touch with a qualified menopause specialist who is at least open-minded about hormone therapy. Numerous women have told me that they've done their own research and are comfortable starting (if not desperately seeking) MHT, yet they get dismissed by their doctors, whose responses range from "Your symptoms are just a part of midlife and you can learn to live with them" to "I don't believe in hormone therapy because we were taught its risks outweigh its benefits."

I do recognize this ignorance or reluctance is not necessarily providers' fault. "I don't blame my doctors who didn't tell me about menopause," shared Dr. Shieva Ghofrany, an OB/GYN and ovarian cancer survivor. "They were trying to keep me alive and didn't have the time or training to go into all that. Our healthcare system is set up so that we learn how to treat things reactively, not to help a healthy person stay healthy."

Indeed, our healthcare providers have not been properly trained. In 2018, Dr. JoAnn Pinkerton, who was then the executive director of what is now The Menopause Society, described to *AARP Magazine*: "'Do most practicing [OB/GYNs] have sufficient nuanced knowledge about menopause and how to treat its symptoms?... I don't think so.'"[31]

The years that followed did not seem to reflect much of an improvement. In 2019, the Mayo Clinic released a study of a survey sent to post-graduate-level trainees in family medicine, internal medicine, and obstetrics and gynecology at US residency programs; the results indicated important gaps in knowledge, particularly as related to the safety of hormone therapy, and reported that only "6.8% felt adequately prepared to manage women experiencing menopause."[32] A 2022 national survey of program directors of OB/GYN residency programs revealed that the majority (about two-thirds!) of programs lacked a dedicated menopause curriculum, and there was a desire and need for more.[33]

If the doctors who specifically study and treat women's reproductive health are not getting enough (or any!) training on this major health transition that impacts about half the population for about one-third of their lives, what does that mean for the women themselves?

It means they must share knowledge they've gained and demand better.

It's pretty evident that better messaging around menopause is needed, including among professionals. The Menopause Society agrees. Its medical director, Dr. Stephanie Faubion, said in September 2024: "Unfortunately, we have not seen HT use increase in the two decades since the publication of the WHI trial results. In fact, usage rates remain under 4 percent [across different age groups], even in women under the age of 60 years who are typically the most symptomatic. These findings suggest that substantial barriers to HT use remain, and additional efforts are needed to educate women and clinicians about menopause management and HT use more specifically."[34]

And while I want to give media and medical institutions the benefit of the doubt, I do believe this trend is largely due to long-standing and deep-rooted misogyny. Brittany Barreto, PhD, a millennial scientist and entrepreneur known as the "Voice of FemTech" who is also the author of *Unlocking Women's Health: FemTech and the Quest for Women's Equity*, explained: "Females have been underrepresented in medical research,* partly because we've had a historical understanding that females are complicated—a sexist mindset, whether intentional or not. This has been the paradigm for research that no one really questioned. But because of this model, we haven't had sufficient data on efficacy of treatment options or preventative measures on women." This of course impacts issues specific to women, like menopause. "Imagine if men went through menopause?!" mused Dr. Alexis Melnick, a millennial reproductive endocrinologist and professor of obstetrics and gynecology at Weill Cornell in New York City. I think we can all accurately assume there would be a lot more data and resources.

Author Angela Garbles put it eloquently in *The Guardian* in 2024: "A lack of definitive information, especially when it comes to female reproductive health, does not indicate that a condition is too obtuse or mysterious to understand. Most likely it means that the condition has been dismissed, undervalued, and poorly researched."[35] Menopause *has* been researched, with experts in agreement that individualized assessments of risks and benefits for patients are the most appropriate approach to treatment and that MHT should be considered, as it is generally safe and effective.[36] And yet, the women who suffer because of it are still too often dismissed, in part because their providers remain underinformed.

---

* In fact, women of reproductive age were generally not included in clinical research until 1993! Read more about the history of excluding women—and the cost of doing so—here: Sandra Rose Salathe, "Why Are Women Still Underrepresented in Clinical Trials?" *Flow Space*, May 15, 2024, https://www.theflowspace.com/physical-health/prevention-longevity/women-underrepresented-in-health-research-2945245.

PROVIDERS ARE SEEKING OUT THEIR OWN TRAINING

Accordingly, healthcare providers have had to take it upon themselves to learn more about menopause. Dr. Caroline Messer, the endocrinologist, recalled: "I fell in love with endocrinology as a medical student at the Mount Sinai School of Medicine. But, we learned very little about menopause during training. I acquired my expertise through conferences and studying the field post-training."

Dr. Mandelberger also proactively sought out her education in this area, after receiving her medical degree from Tufts, completing a residency in Obstetrics and Gynecology at the Mount Sinai Hospital in New York City, and undergoing fellowship training in minimally invasive gynecologic surgery. While practicing gynecology in a corporate health system, she described, "Many of my patients were over 40 and complaining of various symptoms that I thought reflected normal aging—because I had not learned a thing about menopause. Once I realized my gap in knowledge, and the gap in the healthcare system, I delved into the information and made it my mission to help women dealing with these issues." She pursued further training with The Menopause Society to become the certified expert she is today.

Dr. Rebbecca Hertel is an osteopathic physician and certified menopause practitioner who also felt compelled to seek further education in this field. Trained in family medicine, she found herself struggling in her mid-40s with symptoms like irregular periods, hot flashes, mood changes, and significant brain fog. "I felt really scared. I found myself looking at a chart and unable to process what I was reading." Despite her education and experience, she did not immediately recognize what was happening to her. "I had my last child at nearly 40, and my providers indicated my symptoms were just due to being postpartum. One told me that I simply couldn't multitask any more at my age and to accept that."

Well, she didn't accept it. Dr. Hertel pursued her own higher education on menopause. She immersed herself in the courses available by providers like Dr. Corinne Menn and Dr. Heather Hirsch, whose social media and training platforms are discussed further in the next chapter. "My insight into this changed my career," she noted. "I have now devoted my life to helping other women through the menopause transition."

Sarah Shealy is a registered nurse, nurse midwife, and menopause specialist who had a similar experience. "I had years of experience in women's health and despite multiple appointments with experienced healthcare providers, no one ever mentioned I might be in perimenopause," she recounted. Ultimately, she took her health into her own hands by engaging in extensive research, including by reading the primary source literature and learning from professional organizations like The Menopause Society.

"We must self-advocate," affirmed Anne Fulenwider, the Alloy cofounder. "Baby boomers should be pissed their agency was taken away following the 2002 WHI study. Gen X members have said, 'What the fuck?' and are now talking about it and creating solutions like telehealth offerings from providers who are actually trained in menopause care. My hope is that by the time all millennials are in menopause, safe and effective treatment, which may include MHT, will be just as accessible as buying tampons."

My friend Susan Frankel, a healthcare attorney, shares that mindset. She told her story of feeling lost throughout her menopause transition in the anthology book (to which we each contributed chapters), *Own Your Story: Empower. Connect. Create Change.* Frankel's menopause transition has involved mental health struggles, surgically induced menopause following the removal of her ovaries, and multiple phases of trial and error with menopausal hormone therapy regimens. Two different OB/GYNs she saw throughout her 40s never mentioned menopause. Other women in her life who have access to healthcare like she does have similarly been dismissed for their symptoms. "I want women to be informed so that they are not blindsided by what could happen to them and their health, like I was," she explained of sharing.

A NEW GENERATION OF HEALTHCARE

Fortunately, the medical community continues to make strides, especially since a deeper dive into the data has highlighted many pitfalls of the WHI trial. Dr. Messer summarized the main issues of the 2002 WHI research have been identified as follows:

"1. The progesterone used at that time of the trial may have independently led to an increased risk in breast cancer. Women in the trial who did not require progesterone (those who had already had hysterectomies) did not show the same increased risk of breast cancer. We now use a different type of progesterone.

2. The trial analyzed women of all ages in one lump sum. A subgroup analysis performed after the fact showed that newly menopausal women did not have the same risks from hormone replacement therapy as older women.

3. The newly widespread use of estrogen through the skin (in the form of patches or gels) greatly mitigates the risk of blood clots."

The WHI itself has since clarified its 2002 warnings. In 2013, it released a follow-up study, about which Dr. JoAnn Manson, a lead investigator of the Women's Health Initiative and a professor at the Harvard School of Public Health and Harvard Medical School, among other accolades, informed *NPR* that the WHI had never intended to deny hormone therapy to those in early menopause; [37] of the follow-up research, she explained, "The key point is that results are now broken down by age and time since menopause. This is really what women and their clinicians have needed in order to interpret the findings and provide individualized care."[38]

In 2018, Dr. Manson further emphasized to *AARP Magazine*: "'The fragmentation of women's healthcare has led to untreated symptoms and a serious impact on women's health. Many women who would have benefited from hormone therapy may have suffered needlessly."[39] In 2024, Dr. Manson coauthored a new study based on follow-up data from the WHI trial that found that benefits of MHT generally outweigh the risks, especially for younger midlife women. She has said, very clearly, "The [2002] WHI findings should never be used as a reason to deny hormone therapy to women in early menopause with bothersome menopause symptoms."[40]

While the WHI investigators have been busy (but perhaps too quietly) clarifying, many healthcare providers (though not nearly enough, as we've just discussed) have been doing additional research and dedicating themselves to providing comprehensive care to mitigate the fragmentation of women's healthcare. For example, Dr. Alicia Robbins founded her boutique women's health practice in order to provide personalized guidance to women. Modern practice, she told me, is very different from the way our mothers were (or weren't) treated. "Now we usually prescribe FDA-approved bioidentical (vs. synthetic) hormones, which are not shown to increase breast cancer risk (the version of progesterone featured in the 2002 WHI study is generally not prescribed anymore). Now we know that when someone has a uterus, we must give them appropriate dosages of progesterone *and* estrogen, to avoid increased endometrial (uterine) cancer risk from estrogen-HT alone. Now," she confirmed, "we know that perimenopause is complex, nuanced, and can and should be treated with regular check-ups and tweaking, to adjust treatment as women's symptoms adjust."

Now we have more information, including the consensus among menopause specialists that menopausal hormone therapy is generally safe and effective and should be offered as an option to a patient, who should be able to use her agency to make a choice about whether to pursue it.

Once I learned this fact, I was curious what our mothers, after years of hearing a different message, thought of it. When I asked several women of the Baby Boomer generation about hormone therapy, answers ranged. Most were entirely unaware of the updates in research. Accordingly, many were still apprehensive or resistant.

"I didn't want to try any of that, and I still wouldn't." (Sure, that's your choice. But could it be worth learning about, to understand all options? If not for you, for the younger women in your life?) "I would really need to dig into the research to learn about the risks before I made that kind of choice." (Totally get it, you should dig into the research, much of which is cited here, to learn and make a decision that's personal and right for you. And please keep in mind that peer-reviewed pieces from credible academic journals are ideal sources, though there may not be one right answer to your question, especially if it's specific to you. We too often tend to read one source or even one sentence and assume it's applicable to all. We certainly can't do that with menopause!)

I feel sorry for the many women who didn't get the opportunity to try treatments or learn more back in the 2000s and 2010s. Instead they were just denied information and had choices made for them. In so many ways, they were stripped of their autonomy when it came to their reproductive health.

Let's not let that happen to us. As is the case with many other milestones (the right to vote, the right to have one's own line of credit, the right to participate in politics and policymaking, and more), newer generations of women can benefit from and build on the advocacy of previous generations. Let's learn from our mothers, including from what they didn't learn.

HOW CAN MILLENNIALS PREPARE?

Talk to Your Mother (and Keep Talking)

We already know more than our mothers did, but it's also never too late to learn more. If you can, ask your mom about her experience with menopause, including perimenopause. Ask her when her symptoms started, what was helpful for her, and what she would do differently if she could.

And keep talking. Menopause should not be treated as some shameful secret that makes women afraid to ask for help. We have to normalize it—among ourselves, within our homes, and with those who take care of us (or should). "Everyone's menopause journey is unique. But the one commonality I recognize now that my peers and I have been through it," my 70-year-old family friend Vicki told me, "is that whatever your individual experience, you are better off when you talk about it. Everyone needs support, so don't be afraid to be open—open to sharing your journey and open to asking questions and learning about different treatment options."

When women talk about what we are going through, we demand attention to it. Menopausal women like our mothers have been underserved. We know from research and lived experiences that still today, women are struggling to be heard, to get a proper diagnosis for their menopause-related symptoms, or to find healthcare providers who are willing or able to provide the help they need.[41] It takes diligence and inner strength (and patience, I know!) to advocate for yourself in the American healthcare system. But trust in yourself and get support to do so, if you need it. Remember that you are the one who knows your own body best; it's up to you to care for it how you see fit.

Ask More Questions

I believe—I hope—the tide is turning for the better, albeit slowly. It used to be, Dr. Robbins explains, that the medical field thought of menopause (i.e., that official one-year-post-final-menstrual-period mark) as the time to start treatment, but that's false. "If your doctor is telling you that nothing can be done to alleviate symptoms before you reach actual menopause," she said, "it's time to find a new doctor."[42]

Indeed, as my own mother has always advised me: "If you don't ask, you won't get."

So, speak up—even if, based on your mother's experience, you may be years away from your last period. Speak up—even if your periods are regular for you but you've started to feel unlike yourself, if you're suddenly experiencing interrupted sleep, or if you're experiencing hot flash symptoms that your doctor is dismissing because you aren't of a certain age. Speak up—even if hormone therapy isn't for you, but you want information on all possible options, and because you deserve to have it.

Speak up because our mothers felt that they couldn't, and too many women suffered in silence instead. Speak up so that we millennials can get the care we need and deserve. Speak up so that our daughters will have more options than us all.

Chapter 4

MENOPAUSE IN THE MEDIA

Since our mothers didn't teach us much about menopause, many millennials have relied on the media to get some kind of information. But as with most depictions of women and women's issues in mainstream media, representation (and lack thereof) of menopausal women leaves a lot to be desired.

"Everything I have ever known about menopause until about five years ago was from sitcom punchlines about hot flashes," reflected Jo Piazza, the best-selling novelist of *The Sicilian Inheritance* and host of the *Under the Influence* podcast about social media and the ways in which aspirational marketing particularly affects women and mothers. The 1980-born journalist who has decades of experience working in media remembers "menopause getting played for laughs in a very superficial way."

I relate. I consume a lot (and I mean, a lot!) of media targeted toward millennial female audiences and yet could think of only one character who had a relevant storyline: Samantha Jones in the original HBO series *Sex and the City*. (If there are other characters or storylines that come to mind for you, please let me know!)

In the eighth episode of season three, which aired back in 2000 (when Kim Cattrall, the actress who plays her, was about 44), Samantha is offended to receive a catalog for premenopausal women. Her friends grimace and joke sarcastically while discussing treatments and perimenopause (though they don't use that term). They do acknowledge the relief that will come from no longer having to worry about their periods but largely treat menopause as something they fear because it signifies they are old. In fact, the theme of the whole episode is the passage of time. Samantha is seen rolling up her neck skin and crying about "drying up" before we hear a tick-tock clock sound in the musical score.

In the show, Samantha ultimately gets her period, but by the theatrical release of *Sex and the City 2* in 2010, the character seems to have embraced her new life phase. "Very soon you will thank me," she says to Carrie and Miranda. "I am leading the way through the menopause maze with my vitamins, my melatonin sleep patches, my bioidentical estrogen cream, progesterone cream, a touch of testosterone …" Given where we were as a culture at this time (i.e., terrified of HRT following that 2002 WHI study), Samantha, as usual, is notably confident and cool. "I am!" she proudly agrees when called the hormone whisperer. "I've tricked my body into thinking it's younger [...] no hot flashes, no mood swings, my sex drive is right back to where it was."

I love the empowerment reflected in this scene, and I appreciate the growth Samantha shows regarding aging. The *SATC* ladies helped raise me. They taught us all lots of important lessons, including how to feel good in your body and sexuality (and of course, how important female friendship is). But really, Hollywood, shouldn't there be more on menopause?

"Our society devalues older women," proffered Kara Alaimo, the communications professor and *Over the Influence* author. "It's distinct from other cultures, like in Asia, where people revere the elderly. But in the United States, our society lionizes youth and beauty. We see this in Hollywood, in the roles 'older' female actors play—or don't play. Topics that affect older women, like menopause, simply don't get enough coverage in the media, including in the news."

We know that representation matters, and our inability to see midlife women reflected on screen (or in books or on the stage or covered by journalists) has profound implications, not least of which is that our fear of menopause gets perpetuated because it remains such an unknown. Men of a certain age do not face the same challenges. Instead, men's health issues tend to be normalized in the media. In fact, former US Senator and 1996 US presidential candidate Bob Dole appeared on a 1998 television commercial (the drug's first) for Viagra, the erectile dysfunction medication. He spoke directly about the health issue, creating a sense of normalcy around discussing usually private topics, even if it was initially a bit awkward.

Think about how we now perceive Viagra compared with menopause treatments, or to menopause itself. "Menopause is a major turning point in a woman's life and it has been treated like something taboo. On the flipside, when men can't get an erection, they are immediately delivered a drug to fix it. Women should be given the same level of care," Piazza encouraged.

These are all reproductive healthcare issues, yet as a culture, we are more comfortable communicating about—and caring for—men's issues. And the inherent misogyny behind this trend impacts more than the media; it drives medical research as well. "It feels like the medical community doesn't know, and maybe doesn't care, much about women's bodies. There's a long history of medical tests being done on men and assuming the results will be the same for women, even though we clearly know that women's bodies are very different," Alaimo described, referencing research discussed in Caroline Criado Perez's book *Invisible Women: Exposing Data Bias in a World Designed for Men.*

One study, Alaimo shared, particularly stood out to her and is, perhaps unsurprisingly, related to menstruation. Guess what drug seemed to provide considerable relief for women experiencing period pain? That's right, Viagra. But it isn't offered to women and is instead well known as a men's drug for sexual function. Why? Because the trial on women's pain ran out of money, women's issues remain inadequately funded in medical research, and the way men's health is portrayed in the media is incredibly biased, exacerbating a cycle in which women are perpetually missing out on care.

Fortunately, we may be at a turning point. "I think we are at the beginning of growing comfortable with discussing menopause," observed Alaimo. "For example, I feel like everyone around me has been talking about the 2024 novel *Sandwich* by Catherine Newman." (She's not alone; the book was an instant *New York Times* bestseller, among other accolades, and has been the subject of more than one book club in which I participate.) The novel's protagonist is a woman spending time with both her young adult kids and aging parents and, per Alaimo, includes a "very blunt description of menopause. While it's a hilarious and beautifully written book, I also think women are rallying around it because there is an appetite among women at this age, at midlife, to feel more recognized and seen."

Piazza is one such woman ready for more. She is glad to see new, nuanced portrayals in the media. "The monologue in *Fleabag* blew my mind for its raw honesty and completely fresh perspective on menopause," she shared, referring to the third episode of the British comedy's second season, which aired in 2019. In it, the main character has a conversation with her 58-year-old colleague who says with a wry smile: "Women are born with pain ... We have pain on a cycle for years and years and years, and then, just when you feel you are making peace with it all, what happens? The menopause comes!... And it is *the* most wonderful fucking thing in the world ... Then you're free!... It is horrendous, but then it's magnificent. Something to look forward to."

And maybe we can all look forward to more menopause in the media, as it becomes more mainstream. In 2024, even the Kardashians kept up with (or perhaps influenced us to be) growing comfortable with discussing menopause. During season five of their Hulu reality show, *The Kardashians*, the family's matriarch Kris Jenner undergoes surgery to remove her ovaries and uterus upon the recommendation of her doctor because of a tumor. "No one talks about getting older, no one talks about menopause. No one told me about menopause," Kris relays to her girlfriends in episode eight. They reassure her that it's OK to be emotional about the loss of her reproductive organs that helped her have six children who may all be considered millennial icons.

Let's keep building on this media momentum. If you are an author, a producer, a screenwriter, an actor, a radio show host, a media personality, or simply a consumer of media, keep pushing for more depictions of menopause. Keep sharing and celebrating those characters, storylines, and conversations. And as you're doing so, keep reminding yourself: You're doing amazing, sweetie.

HOW CAN MILLENNIALS PREPARE?

Demand Better Media Portrayals

We must demand more realistic, accurate portrayals of women in all media, when it comes to menopause and beyond. Even the gorgeous Golden Bachelorette,* Joan Vassos, has said she felt invisible upon getting older.[43] It's (past) time to see these women, perhaps starting on our screens!

---

* Yes I am a loyal fan of the TV franchise. Fellow pit-dwellers, get in touch.

Women consistently consume more media than men.[44] We are an influential audience! We must call out gender biases, ageism, and all forms of discrimination. We must share diverse and subtly complex depictions of midlife women with each other and with all people (no matter gender or age) in our life. We must write about and amplify women's stories in order to normalize our experiences and attain much-needed education.

Consume and Share Accurate Media

Since you are reading this book, you already appreciate traditional media as a source of information (even if it's on a device, it counts, yay!). I recommend other nonfiction from leading experts of the current menopause movement, including *Grown Woman Talk: Your Guide to Getting and Staying Healthy,* by Sharon Malone, MD (who is particularly passionate about empowering women of color with knowledge and agency), *The Menopause Brain: New Science Empowers Women to Navigate the Pivotal Transition with Knowledge and Confidence,* by Lisa Mosconi, PhD (a leading neuroscientist and women's brain health specialist who presents data, anecdotes, and guidance on the ways estrogen decline affects the brain), and *The New Menopause: Navigating Your Path Through Hormonal Change with Purpose, Power, and Facts,* by Mary Claire Haver, MD (who provides advice to women on how to speak with their healthcare providers about midlife wellness, among other incredibly important nuggets of knowledge).

If you prefer to watch or listen to your media, consider these platforms:

- *Health by Heather Hirsch* podcast with Dr. Heather Hirsch

  Dr. Heather Hirsch is not only a physician who treats women in multiple states through her telemedicine practice, but also an educator on everything peri/menopause. The podcast features interviews with additional experts on topics ranging from painful sex to heart health and is just one of her robust offerings; others include her Instagram account (@heatherhirschmd), her comprehensive website including her free guide to hormones, her training courses for both laypersons and healthcare providers (I'm an appreciative student!), her YouTube channel, and her book, *Unlock Your Menopause Type: Personalized Treatments, the Last Word on Hormones, and Remedies That Work.*

- *Dr. Streicher's Inside Information: THE Menopause Podcast* with Dr. Lauren Streicher

  Dr. Lauren Streicher is the founding medical director of the Northwestern Medicine Center for Sexual Medicine and Menopause. Dr. Streicher is also a regular media contributor and best-selling author of numerous books on women's health. She serves on the editorial board of The Menopause Society's journal, *Menopause*. Her podcast explores all sorts of menopause symptoms, answering questions you may not have ever asked out loud, and delves into the latest myths and misinformation to clarify for and empower the listener.

- **Let's Talk Menopause**

  Let's Talk Menopause is a nonprofit that provides free and important monthly virtual talks with leading experts via its website LetsTalkMenopause.org. Cofounded by fellow social worker Donna Klassen, LCSW, the organization's mission is to advocate for the medical community to invest in menopause healthcare, educate the public, and empower and connect women for support through menopause. The talks—which are among other programs it offers, alongside public awareness campaigns and a podcast—cover topics women want to learn more about, including the cognitive effects of the menopause transition and stories from Black women and the doctors who listened to them.

- **Mama Beasts**

  Virtual events are organized by the media brand Mama Beasts. Live online gatherings and their recordings are available at MamaBeasts.com, on topics including Perimenopause 101 (I'm featured) and Perimenopause Bootcamp: Fitness & Nutrition Musts. Mama Beasts founder Antoinette Hemphill said of her reason for sharing: "It's important to get loud about perimenopause through our community and content because women tend to be too quiet everywhere else in their lives, careful not to inconvenience anyone or complain too much even when we know our health is suffering. We tend to take large systematic failures and internalize them, finding ways to blame ourselves even when we know better." She believes that honest and real conversations about our health enable women to discuss hard things in an unfiltered way. "And with vulnerability comes connection—and power."

- **Perry: Perimenopause Community**

  This app and digital wellness platform is designed to build community among women in perimenopause, featuring various webinars and group chat opportunities on topics like perimenopause treatment for breast cancer survivors. Among the platform's best resources are its symptom tracker checklist and its journal/handbook, which contains contributions from a wide range of menopause specialists. Health providers and other specialists can be trained in holistic perimenopause care through the new Perry Care hub. In December 2024, Perry released a Perimenopause Trend Report available for download on its website, heyperry.com, which contains important insight from analysis of two hundred thousand conversations about perimenopause from its users that year.

- *Thriving Through Perimenopause* **YouTube series with Dr. Anna Glezer**
  The founder of Women's Wellness Psychiatry, Dr. Anna Glezer runs a virtual practice based in the San Francisco area, and the Reproductive & Integrative Psychiatry fellowship program, which I have participated in to receive advanced training in women's mental health. Dr. Glezer is board certified in adult and forensic psychiatry and is passionate about helping as many women as possible through her direct services and media contributions related to reproductive mental health. She provides many educational offerings like webinars for clinicians and this six-part free video series on perimenopause, which includes menopause myths, symptoms, and treatment options.

- *You Are Not Broken* **podcast with Dr. Kelly Casperson**
  Dr. Kelly Casperson is a urologist whose mission is to teach women about sex and empower them to create a better life while feeling less alone. The podcast offers practical information in a relatable tone, focusing on women in midlife and featuring expert guests on topics like what couples should know about hormones

and how they may impact libido and embracing humor and fun while dating in midlife. Dr. Casperson's book, *You Are Not Broken*, and her virtual courses are also topnotch resources for adult sex education.

And of course, as millennials, we are digital natives. We are powerful through our social media use. We entered adulthood on Facebook and Instagram, and even though those platforms might be cheugy, we still love them. Studies repeatedly show that the majority of millennials spend hours on social media daily.[45] While I often have mixed feelings about social media use, one positive outcome is that formerly unmentionable topics have become mainstream. Upon a quick social media search, you'll be able to find influencers on various apps, even the professional social network LinkedIn, posting about menopause.

These Instagram platforms (TikTok is beyond my skillset as an elder millennial, let's be real) are amazing, accessible ways to learn and share information:

- @aliciarobbinsmd
  Dr. Alicia Robbins has a bedside manner that makes her approachable to all who check out her page. A fellow millennial mom, she makes scientific content easy to understand, sharing information on topics like menopausal weight gain, vaginal probiotics, and more, citing data and anecdotal experience.

- @drjaynemorgan
  Dr. Jayne Morgan is a cardiologist and the executive director of health and community education at the Piedmont Healthcare

Corporation in Atlanta. Through her account, she shares her numerous media appearances and webinars discussing important issues for midlife women, including cholesterol, disparities in menopause care, and cardiovascular disease risk for Black women.

- @drmandelberger

  Dr. Adrienne Mandelberger is the gynecologic surgeon who founded Balanced Medical and All Things Menopause, an educational resource for women's health in midlife and beyond. On social media, she shares relatable content on everything from fibroids (which, I learned from her, are very common benign tumors of the uterus that may require surgery if causing pain or other problems) to *Fraggle Rock* (as in, if you recognize the characters from this iconic '80s puppet TV show, it's time for you to learn about perimenopause).

- @drrachelrubin

  Dr. Rachel Rubin is a urologist and sexual medicine specialist based in the DC area. Her enthusiasm for educating women and providing patient-centered care is evident through Instagram as well as her YouTube channel (where she focuses on menopausal genitourinary symptoms and often refers to vaginal hormones as nonnegotiable) and volunteer work (she is the former education chair and current director-at-large for ISSWSH, the International Society for the Study of Women's Sexual Health).

- @drsalaswhalen

  Dr. Rocio Salas-Whalen is an endocrinologist passionate about changing the narrative around women's health and obesity. A triple board-certified and bilingual (English/Spanish) physician

based in New York City, she provides information and resources on topics including how drugs for weight loss and diabetes (known as semaglutide, tirzepatide, and/or GLP-1 medications) can assist with wellness goals during midlife.

- @gynogirl

  Dr. Sameena Rahman is a gynecologist and women's health specialist at the Center for Gynecology and Cosmetics in Chicago. She serves on the board of numerous organizations, including ISSWSH. Through social media, Dr. Rahman breaks down the latest menopause-related research and presents information on orgasms, libido, painful sex (sex should not be painful!), and more in relatable ways.

- @hotpausehealth

  HotPause Health is a community seeking to empower and connect women in peri/menopause through science-backed resources and a little bit of humor. Their platform includes resources on legislation affecting midlife women's health, nutrient-rich recipes from women's health experts, and clear information on various forms of menopausal treatment.

- @jackie.giannellinptalks

  Jackie Giannelli is a certified family nurse practitioner licensed in CA, CT, FL, MA, NV, and NY who specializes in women's sexual health. Via her social media, she breaks down scientific research into understandable tips (like demonstrating #girlmath for testosterone) all the while advocating for women's well-being.

- **@menoscandal**

  Journalist Kate Muir from the United Kingdom is the woman behind this account that shares groundbreaking menopause research, news, and pop culture menopause moments. She is also the author of a book, *Everything You Need to Know About the Menopause (but Were Too Afraid to Ask)*, and coproducer of a documentary, *Sex, Myths, and The Menopause*, that are great resources.

- **@tamsenfadal**

  Tamsen Fadal is a journalist who coproduced with Joanne LaMarca Mathisen the documentary *The M Factor* (a must-see that is the first of its kind to offer continuing education credits to medical providers!) and is an all-around incredible resource and menopause advocate. She shares information and experiences related to menopause's impact on mental health, her hormone regimen, her exercise and nutrition routines, and much more.

- **@thisisflowspace**

  I'm a big fan of this account for the online magazine *Flow Space*, which focuses on reproductive health, physical health, mental health, interpersonal health, and style for women of all ages. In particular, I love its features celebrating women over 40!

American women tend to be self-taught about menopause, so it's important that we rely on accurate resources.[46] So, keep consuming (well-vetted) media, and please, keep sharing. Send me an Instagram DM via @thecounselaur to share some of your favorite accounts! I am reading, watching, and listening along with you.

I was delighted to read, for example, about Piazza's experiences with a perimenopausal period and period panties in her Substack newsletter. "The only way that we can change the media around menopause is to share and amplify as many real-life stories as possible through a female lens," she responded, when asked why she felt compelled to share. "I think a lot of media around menopause and the cultural stereotypes have been generated by men. It is time that we take control of our own narrative."

I agree. Thank you for holding, quite literally, my new narrative.

Chapter 5

FROM PREGNANCY TO PERIMENOPAUSE

• •

Something magical happened to me when I became a mom, and it had little to do with the baby. It had to do with the women in my life. Women who had been friends of mine for decades and women I met fleetingly, for a few moments, whose names I didn't even catch or can't currently remember. Women of every age and generation, reflecting a wide range of cultural backgrounds and races, in various settings that I wouldn't have previously expected to be so open and intimate. With these women, I readily talked about body parts, caregiving decisions, sex, mental health, and more.

I welcomed advice from women who had been where I was before. "Oh, are your breasts hurting, honey? Try to release a little milk manually so you feel better, and we'll get you home as soon as you need," suggested the kind saleswoman at a department store during my first outing away from my little one, when I was desperate for a couple of hours of me-time (and shopping for an outfit for an upcoming family event that I felt good wearing—especially given the swollen boobs which, by the way, tend to get even bigger during pregnancy if you're breastfeeding or pumping—and, I'm told, during menopause, too!). "I loved going straight to formula," my mom's friend recalled of her experiences a generation prior. "It was good for my mental health and my husband's, who got to feed the baby from the bottle and bond."

I was open with women who had different experiences from mine or who had not yet become moms themselves. "Did you poop during labor?" a friend five years younger asked, without hesitation, eager for information on the mystery of childbirth as she considered her own family plans. "You don't have to have sex just because you are 'allowed to,'" advised a woman I met while walking with the baby in the stroller, whose own was a few months older than mine. "It feels really weird and your body is still unlike your own. Don't push yourself. And hold a cold soda can in between your legs after to help with any soreness. It felt good for me, and I didn't even have a vaginal birth!"

It became clear to me that there was something about motherhood, including among those not yet mothers, that women just *got*. It felt comforting to know that when I said, "I had a baby a few months ago," a stranger could understand the layers of emotions and logistics that I was navigating. A woman I didn't know at all could say, "It's OK to cry," and mean it.

In many ways, motherhood neutralizes us all, a fact I'm reminded of frequently. I was reminded when the confident girl who intimidated me in middle school called me crying from sleep deprivation and overwhelm, looking for advice on childcare for her newborn. I was reminded when I saw the chic woman in my extended social circle who always seemed put together eat dinner off her kids' plates while standing up, worrying about whether they were being excluded from their friend group, just like we all do.

Once I became a mom, I felt like I could trust other women, sometimes without even having to say anything at all. I felt like I was taken care of by other women, so much so that I ultimately chose to focus my career on taking care of other women and moms because I wanted to share that experience. And while this happened to me upon becoming a mother, I believe that women in general, whether or not they are mothers or want to be, can share such a bond if they're open to it.

I've noticed similar energy when it comes to issues like safety or security in various forms. Women will say, "Let me know when you get home," because we know the range of bullshit women have to endure while walking alone, even in safe cities in the middle of the day. Women will readily share recommendations for medical specialists, financial advisers, or divorce attorneys with other women, because we know that it's important to work with professionals who really understand what women need. Women will share their wisdom to support other women, even if it means sharing something really private.

Millennials have been doing so for years in the context of fertility challenges, but it hasn't always been this way. "I had 'unexplained infertility,' a term I had never even heard of before I was diagnosed with it," revealed my millennial friend Alexis Cirel, a law partner who focuses on fertility and family law in New York. "Fertility challenges tend to be stigmatized and kept private, which leads to shame, isolation, and ignorance—you don't know what you don't know, and often you don't even know where to begin when you're trying to learn more. But I believe knowledge is power."

Cirel spoke with countless fertility experts, other doctors, and women who had been where she was before so she could get educated and make informed choices. "Once I realized there was a gap in policy, I took the lead on helping change the law in my state to allow for gestational surrogacy and make it more of an accessible option to struggling families." Now a mother of two, she shares the knowledge she gained with other women and families going through fertility challenges.

And it should be known that potential options regarding fertility can be complex and potentially limited as women approach menopause. I realize it may come as a shock to think about perimenopause if you're still thinking (or haven't even yet thought) about procreating, but it's important to understand why women might have to.

"It feels like I'm in a race against time," a friend born in 1982 once told me. She was a mom of two by the time her 40th birthday arrived, a big milestone she didn't feel like celebrating. She was in the midst of trying to get pregnant with her desperately desired third child.

"I know it'll get harder as I age, yet obviously I can't press pause on getting older."

Generally, we consider aging better than its alternative. But as a culture, we still tend to fear it. For women, especially those who want to have children, menopause can be a particularly scary part of aging because it explicitly marks the end of an era: that of fertility.

"Menopause is the depletion of the eggs left in a woman's ovaries," explained Lilli Dash Zimmerman, a board-certified OB/GYN and fertility specialist at Northwell Health on Long Island, New York. Added Taraneh Nazem, a double board-certified reproductive endocrinologist and fertility specialist and OB/GYN at RMA of New York: "Women are born with all the eggs they will ever have in their ovaries—which, at birth, is about 1 to 2 million. By the time a female has her first period, she is down to 300,000 to 500,000 eggs on average. The majority of those eggs will never be used." This is basically what we are referring to when we use terms like "a woman's biological clock"—and partly why our society is very fearful of aging.

So, what happens as we get older and closer to menopause? "Generally, by a woman's 40s, the quality of eggs drastically declines in terms of chromosomal make-up. So, the best predictor of a successful pregnancy is female age, regardless of ovarian reserve (i.e., number of eggs)," Dr. Zimmerman elaborated. "Because of egg quality, a woman in her 20s or early 30s who has a low ovarian reserve has a better chance of a successful pregnancy than a woman in her mid-40s with a high ovarian reserve. It's more about quality, not quantity—though as aforementioned, the number of eggs is also naturally decreasing as we age."

It is still absolutely possible to have a healthy pregnancy while in one's 40s. It's also increasingly common. Today, women in the United States are becoming mothers later in life than in previous decades,[47] with more than a hundred thousand Americans in their 40s giving birth each year.[48] Dr. Zimmerman confirmed, "You can definitely get pregnant while you're in perimenopause." In fact, data show that about a third of pregnancies among women 40 or older are unplanned.[49] I frequently hear statements like "My period wasn't regular, so I assumed I wasn't ovulating," or "I had trouble getting pregnant with my other kids so I assumed at this age it would be next to impossible—I assumed wrong!" Dr. Zimmerman clarified: "The likelihood of pregnancy is lower than it was before perimenopause, but the bottom line is that as long as you are ovulating and sperm meets eggs at time of ovulation, there is a chance of pregnancy."

Of course, if you don't want to take that chance and become pregnant, you should use a form of birth control (or contraception) until you officially hit menopause, no matter how irregular or infrequent your periods become as you age. The combination birth control pill (or "oral contraceptive") is one way to prevent pregnancy. Per Dr. Zimmerman, "The pill does not affect ovarian reserve and it does not affect or delay menopause. What the pill does is prevent ovulation, in addition to providing other potential benefits (including menopause symptom relief) that each woman should address with her healthcare provider." Dr. Nazem confirmed: "The pill can be a really beautiful thing, not just for preventing pregnancy but also for alleviating symptoms like acne or painful cramps from endometriosis, fibroids, or other gynecologic problems. It does *not* impact fertility long-term."

What about the women who do want to get pregnant and are closer to menopause than puberty, like my 40-year-old friend (who did, eventually, have a beautiful baby through in vitro fertilization)? "There are still many options for women as they age," reassured Dr. Zimmerman. "About half of my patients are in their 40s. They seek fertility care to better monitor or induce ovulation, decrease risk of chromosomal abnormalities, and utilize various assisted reproductive technologies like the use of frozen embryos or donor eggs (more common than you might think), which they can still carry since the uterus does not age the same way the ovaries do."

OK, so let's say you're a millennial who is hoping to have kids soon (whether your first or your fourth) and you're concerned about your egg quality. Or maybe you had children in the last decade and are feeling like your body is just becoming recognizable as your own again. And now here I am, telling you to get ready for menopause. You're probably thinking: *Hey now, this is NOT what dreams are made of*—and I understand!

From a psychological perspective, it can be a big adjustment to go from pregnant to perimenopausal, which many millennials will do in a short amount of time. "We *just* finished having babies!" a friend born in 1981 expressed. "I feel like I'm finally getting into a groove as a young mom, and now, suddenly, my body is telling me that I'm a middle-aged woman?" Another friend, who was born in 1989, shared: "My body changed so much during my fertility issues and pregnancies. It's been a few years since I was last postpartum and I am still trying to get back to my pre-baby body. But now I'm experiencing night sweats and brain fog. Will the changes ever end?!"

Women today are having babies later than they used to for a variety of reasons, which can mean that they are closer to perimenopause while postpartum without even realizing it.[50] In fact, I've spoken to quite a few women who had children at 39 or 40 and shortly after began their menopause transition. "When my third baby was about a year old and I was 41, I started experiencing wild mood swings, really up and down and all over the place. I thought I was going crazy," shared a family friend who was born in 1953. "My periods had also gotten clumpier, my skin changed, and I started getting hot flashes. My gynecologist recognized it as perimenopause. I really believe that male doctors would have dismissed me as having postpartum depression given my age and the mood symptoms, but I knew, and she confirmed right away, that it wasn't—which thankfully helped me get the right kind of treatment I needed."

How did she know, when the symptoms can overlap, and both the perinatal and perimenopausal phases are times when women may feel really vulnerable? She knew because she had spoken to her mother about her own early menopause. She knew because she had spoken to other women who experienced postpartum mood disorders and other women who had experienced mood swings during perimenopause. She knew because her doctor, a woman, took the time to evaluate her and her health history. She knew because she knew herself, and she knew because of the wisdom of other women.

HOW CAN MILLENNIALS PREPARE?

Recognize Perinatal Plus Perimenopausal

It's confusing that many symptoms of pregnancy and postpartum can overlap with those of perimenopause, including fatigue, mood swings, irregular periods, tender breasts, and changes in weight. Is your teariness due to the baby blues, to fluctuating perimenopausal hormones, something else, or all of the above? Whatever the reason, you deserve recognition and help throughout these stages, and the sooner the better.

Consider the consequences if you do not get adequate assistance. For example, "women experience many pelvic floor changes during pregnancy and childbirth that they too often don't get support for," noted Sara Reardon, a millennial board-certified women's health and pelvic floor therapist, author, and founder of The Vagina Whisperer, a pelvic floor fitness platform. "Then they start perimenopause with pelvic floor functioning at half capacity, potentially leading to exacerbated symptoms of urinary leakage, organ floor prolapse*, or constipation." Dr. Reardon encourages all pregnant and postpartum women to implement pelvic floor rehabilitation exercises, ideally before perimenopause.

Once in perimenopause, though, it's not too late to get pelvic health support. And it's not too late to get pregnant. If you are 35 or older, you should see a fertility specialist for a full work-up, including

---

* Friends, this is when one or more of the organs, like the uterus, bowel, or bladder, basically falls into the vagina, potentially causing pain, a heaviness feeling, discomfort during peeing or sex, etc.—let's avoid it!

blood work and ultrasounds, if you want to learn all your options. "It's always a good idea to map out a plan for the future if you can," reflected Dr. Nazem.

Learn About Family Planning Possibilities

In general, learning about your options as early as possible is key. "Ugh, I can't even think about menopause!" a friend born in 1988 replied when I told her about this book. But I believe we must think about it. And we must talk about it, so that we can learn from each other and feel less lonely wherever we are in our reproductive lifespan or journeys.

As you'll read repeatedly, every woman experiences menopause differently. None of the physicians with whom I spoke had personal knowledge or awareness of research that indicated the menopause transition was different for women who have given birth compared with those who had not, or for women who had experienced fertility struggles compared with those who had not. So, having children is not a predictor of a menopausal experience. That said, if you do want children (or more children), consider what you need to do before menopause to have them, especially if you want to use your own eggs.

If you are a younger millennial and you don't think that you'll have all the kids you want by the time you reach age 35, consider freezing your eggs now. "Oocyte cryopreservation is a wonderful option to preserve optimal quality eggs," explained Dr. Zimmerman. "A woman in her 40s can be considered young in so many ways, she has so much ahead of her—but it's an unfortunate reality that our ovaries have not evolved along with our cultural perception of midlife." If it turns out that your mom went through menopause at an early age, you may especially want to consider fertility-preserving options.

Neither Dr. Zimmerman nor I have ever met a woman who regrets freezing her eggs. Instead, as a therapist who primarily works with women in the perinatal period, I frequently hear reflections like, "I wish I had been taught earlier about egg quality and all the options I could proactively take to build the family I want." Egg freezing and fertility treatments in general can be costly, unfortunately, but the general consensus among specialists and laywomen is: If you can access the financial resources (potentially through your employer), do it.

For older millennials closer to menopause and, as such, the end of fertility, hope is not lost if you want to add to your family. If applicable, you may want to get off the pill and all birth control methods in order to more accurately track your menstrual cycle and any changes to it. "The pill does not actually affect the timing of menopause or overall ovarian reserve. But if you are on it, you may not realize that your cycle has changed, reflecting potential perimenopause, if your 'period' is in fact due to the pill's placebo or if it's nonexistent due to a hormonal IUD," Dr. Zimmerman pointed out.

We must also share and be empathetic to experiences across the age divide. "When I was menopausal and meeting other moms who had babies the same age as my one-year-old, I felt embarrassed," a 1953-born friend shared. "I didn't tell them about it because they would have thought I was a grandma with a toddler and it felt weird. But if I were going through this now, I think I would share. So what if those other, younger moms couldn't quite relate? Everyone has their own struggles, and we all deserve support."

And women who are not mothers deserve support, too. "How dare you say the word 'menopause' to a single woman who doesn't yet have kids?" a 1987-born friend said to me. She was half-joking, but her remarks were significant. It was scary for her to consider the end of her fertility before she had even begun her family. Furthermore, as a culture, we too often judge a woman's value based on her status as a mother (or not). It's time for change.

To the women who are already mothers, to the women who are not yet but one day want to be, and to those who intend to never be pregnant or be a mom—ultimately, you will all go through menopause. The impact your menopausal experience will have on your fertility and family will vary. But you should know that you are not alone, that other women—including those who have had similar experiences and those who have not—will talk with you, teach you, and support you. You should know that you have choices. And I hope that you feel empowered to make them.

Chapter 6

YOUR BODY, YOUR CHOICE(S): MENOPAUSE AND MEDICINE

While we're thinking about choices, let's dig a little deeper into medical treatment options for menopause. At this point in your perimenopause journey (and maybe always), you may be feeling good enough without needing or desiring some kind of medical involvement. Or, you may be really interested in medical treatments and how they may help during this period of life. So let's look at what that medicine for menopause might mean.

By now you know that you have many more options than our mothers did. Today, healthcare providers and women are more readily taking individually tailored approaches, especially since the message of "hormone therapy is unequivocally dangerous for you" following the 2002 WHI study has been effectively debunked.[51]

As a reminder, the most important thing I have learned from my research with dozens of clinicians and medical experts, many of whom are cited in this chapter, and even more women who have been through it is: The menopause transition, including perimenopause and postmenopause, is different for every woman. It is of utmost importance that you receive personalized care for your symptoms that is based on your personal medical history, risk factors, and goals.

"I want women to realize that there are bespoke solutions for each patient," urged Dr. Caroline Messer, the New York-based endocrinologist. Dr. Adrienne Mandelberger, the gynecologic surgeon and menopause specialist, also emphasized a customized approach. "Everyone deserves an unbiased, comprehensive conversation with their informed healthcare provider about all of their menopause-related treatment options," she said.

You're not alone if the idea that there are lots of potential symptom management options makes you feel overwhelmed (I mean, if we *can* ever just be "whelmed," it's unlikely to be now). "Doctors also like clear answers," acknowledged Dr. Mandelberger. "Throughout menopause, the symptoms can be really vague, and potentially attributed to other medical or environmental reasons. But if you take a good interview from a patient, assess where they are in their life and in their cycle, you can find patterns. It often emerges very clearly that the symptoms can be attributed to the menopause transition. And there are safe and effective treatment approaches to those symptoms."

When I personally set out to learn more, I realized many of my questions were shared by other millennials. I admit that I found myself googling basic questions about the endocrine system that I would hope the average American high schooler can answer. Yet discussions with friends confirmed I was far from alone. It became obvious that we all had a lot to learn.

So, let's do it! Since we went through Menopause for Millennials 101 earlier, let's break down the menopause transition and medical treatment options into what I'll call, Menopause for ~~Dummies~~ Smart Women Who Were Never Taught Anything About It & Want to Learn. School is back in session!

MENOPAUSE FOR ~~DUMMIES~~ SMART WOMEN WHO WERE NEVER TAUGHT ANYTHING ABOUT IT & WANT TO LEARN

(Remember! The information herein is not medical advice, but rather information that you should discuss with your healthcare provider in the context of your personal health. As a nonprescriber, I am intentionally not giving information on dosage amounts or many brand names, as these are specifics you should discuss with your provider.)

Why might I want medical treatment for peri/menopause symptoms?

In addition to changes in one's menstrual cycle, other very common perimenopause symptoms include interrupted sleep, changes in mood, hot flashes, and weight gain. Plus, I've come to learn there's a long list of other potential symptoms during the menopause transition that can often impact and exacerbate each other.

Ready? OK! Bring it on ... Symptoms may include:

- Low energy
- Feeling faint or dizzy
- Poor focus and/or other exacerbated attention-deficit/hyperactivity disorder (ADHD) symptoms like difficulty with executive functioning
- Brain fog feelings or loss of memory
- Changes to sense of smell
- Changes in body odor
- Changes to one's allergens and/or allergic reactions because of changes to histamine levels
- Changes to one's voice
- Sensitive gums
- Other dental issues like tooth decay or loss
- Itchy mouth
- Burning mouth
- Experiencing a metallic taste
- Headaches including migraines or head pressure

- Ringing in the ears (tinnitus)
- "Cold flashes" in which one feels an uncomfortable chill
- Urinary urgency or incontinence or other bladder issues
- Itchy anus
- Heartburn
- Heart palpitations
- Difficulty breathing
- Chest pain
- Bloating
- Gastrointestinal issues
- Low libido
- Numbness or a feeling of tingling (like "pins and needles")
- Muscle tension or aches, including "frozen shoulder syndrome"
- Joint inflammation
- Autoimmune disorder symptom flare-ups
- Generally really bad PMS before menstruating
- Periods involving extremely heavy bleeding that I've heard described as monsoons or murder scenes

… and many more. The limit does not exist!

As a psychotherapist, I was particularly humbled to learn that many (up to 70 percent of) perimenopausal women experience a roller coaster of emotions and psychological symptoms, including irritability, rage, low motivation, crying spells, and loss of self-esteem.[52] *Awesome, oh wow, like totally freak me out* is not an inappropriate response to all this information. (We'll discuss mood and mental health much more in Chapter 8.)

To reiterate, however, not every woman experiences all—or any—of these symptoms. And if you are feeling any, other medical issues that could be causing those symptoms must be considered. For example, if your primary concern is fatigue, Dr. Mandelberger would prompt, "Are you sleeping well? And if not, is that because of illness or situational factors?" She explained that it's necessary to rule out those causes, but, "in the absence of anything else, if you have symptoms and it's the right time of your life, we can presume it's perimenopause."

And if it is perimenopause and your symptoms are bothersome, causing you to suffer, or simply making you curious about your next reproductive health stage, you deserve information on your potential medical treatment options.

How should I approach the peri/menopause treatment conversation with my medical provider?

At your annual visits—or *whenever* you are noticing any changes negatively impacting your well-being—bring them up! Maybe you aren't ready for or in need of some kind of medication, but it's worth having a record of what your baseline is and any shifts. And your provider should be aware, too (and rule out alternative explanations, as mentioned above). It is essential that women work with providers who are not only knowledgeable but also compassionate in order to get the right kind of medical treatment (including, potentially, MHT) for their symptoms. Once I started talking to women about the menopause transition, I realized that (way too) many had been dismissed by their doctors, who said (highly inaccurate and ridiculously condescending) things like, "Your symptoms really need to be ruining your life for you to pursue treatment," or "You need to wait till you reach menopause and stop periods to consider medical options for your symptoms," or "You don't seem to be in perimenopause because your blood work appears normal."

In general, hormone blood tests are *not* used as a standard diagnostic tool for perimenopause. In fact, Dr. Mandelberger told me there is no diagnostic checklist or formalized list of criteria for perimenopause, and testing estrogen and progesterone reflects just one moment in a time of many hormonal fluctuations. "Even if your hormones look 'normal,' you still may be in perimenopause," she explained. For someone who appreciates precise plans and straightforward solutions (it's me, hi), such lack of clarity can be frustrating. But, per Dr. Robbins, "The main way we diagnose perimenopause is based on how a woman feels and her history. It's a very individualized diagnosis."

Rebbecca Hertel, DO, agreed. As the founder of Osteopathic Midlife Health, she offers specialized telemedicine services to patients in multiple states and consultations for other patients to bring to local providers. "Perimenopause can be tricky to treat! It absolutely varies from woman to woman. But all women can be helped. You must keep an open line of communication with your menopause specialist and ensure you are somehow recording your symptoms."

All of the menopause specialists I spoke with confirmed that they regularly engage in very comprehensive conversations with their patients to understand any changes to their body or mood and discuss options. And, in line with the latest research and professional guidelines, they all believe in offering education and nuanced conversations about MHT.

What exactly is menopausal hormone therapy (MHT) and how might it help perimenopausal women?

MHT is the umbrella term for medicine that contains hormones like estrogen, progesterone, or testosterone to treat the symptoms of the menopause transition. Though providers are still largely inconsistent with how they use terminology, it's important to clarify MHT vs. HRT. "Hormone *replacement* therapy or 'HRT' is really an accurate term only for women who experience early or premature menopause before age 45, wherein their hormones are being physiologically replaced with doses that are usually higher compared with the MHT given when natural menopause (after age 45) occurs." Dr. Hertel explained. "MHT for natural/spontaneous menopause usually involves relatively low levels of estrogen and/or progesterone—usually lower than a man has!"

During the menopause transition, estrogen and progesterone fluctuate and ultimately decline (progesterone usually declines first), while FSH levels rise. As a result, women can experience the above-listed symptoms (or others). So MHT can be incredibly helpful to alleviate the effects of the hormonal roller coasters. The Menopause Society has explained: "Because the [menopause transition] is marked by hormone instability, providing consistent sex steroid levels can result in multisystem symptom relief. *This strategy is the best first option for women without contraindications for hormones* [emphasis added]."[53] MHT is often called the "gold standard of care" for alleviating menopause symptoms by medical professionals.

At midlife, women's testosterone levels tend to decline as well, so testosterone may also be prescribed on its own or along with estrogen and/or progesterone during perimenopause. "Contrary to cultural rhetoric that associates testosterone with males, testosterone is very much also a female hormone," described Dr. Robbins. For testosterone, lab tests *could* be helpful to determine if levels are low, especially if a woman's clinical symptoms are low libido and fatigue. Dr. Robbins added, "Testosterone can affect and be helpful for sex drive, body composition, brain fog, bone health, energy, and motivation." I have heard from women who take it that it can also help with focus and cognitive clarity, joint inflammation, and strength.

Hormone therapy is currently FDA-approved for the following:[54]

- To treat specific perimenopause and menopause symptoms, including moderate to severe vasomotor symptoms (like hot flashes and night sweats) and genitourinary symptoms (affecting urinary and genital organs);
- To prevent bone loss and fracture (i.e., improve osteopenia, a condition of low bone mineral density not quite meeting osteoporosis diagnostic levels);
- To help women with hypoestrogenism, a condition characterized by low levels of estrogen caused by hypogonadism (in which a woman experiences impaired production of estrogen) or as a result of primary ovarian insufficiency or surgeries like bilateral oophorectomies (where both ovaries are removed). In fact, in

general, for women who have experienced POI or premature or early menopause, hormone therapy is *recommended* at least until the average age of spontaneous menopause (along with screening to detect medical issues and counseling on fertility, mental health, nutrition, and exercise).

Are birth control and MHT related?

If you feel like the last time you thought about estrogen and progesterone via medicine was in the context of birth control, you're not wrong. A birth control pill, for example, can be considered a form of "hormone therapy" itself: the most common kind is a "combination pill" that contains both estrogen and a form of progesterone to prevent pregnancy. Many contraception options involve only progesterone, like a progestin-only birth control pill, implant, injection, or IUD. All of these options help prevent pregnancy and can mask perimenopause symptoms, including changes to one's period (though they do *not* impact the age at which menopause occurs).

A hormonal birth control method can also help alleviate perimenopause symptoms. For example, "the combination pill can help manage some of the torture of the cycle," advised Dr. Mandelberger. "It can help offset the low dips in estrogen leading to mood symptoms like irritability, and its progesterone helps with heavy or irregular bleeding. The pill is often worth trying in early perimenopause when women are still having fairly regular menstrual cycles." I know several millennial women who have shifted from an IUD to a combination birth control pill to help regulate the mood swings they noticed were worsening as they entered their 40s (while still seeking to avoid pregnancy).

If you're a millennial on a form of birth control, how might you know you need a change in hormone treatment? As usual, by self-monitoring your symptoms and by discussing any adjustments with your healthcare provider. Natalie Givargidze, an adult nurse practitioner, advanced practice registered nurse, and certified menopause practitioner, explained: "If you are on oral contraceptives and still experiencing menopause symptoms like hot flashes, night sweats, poor sleep, joint aches/pains, brain fog, and vaginal dryness, it's usually a good indicator you will do better switching over to an MHT regimen."

It may be counterintuitive, but MHT actually contains much *lower* doses of hormones than traditional birth control. The hormones in contraceptives are primarily used to stop ovulation and suppress a woman's own production of fluctuating hormones by providing steadier levels (so, symptoms are managed and cycles are regulated). Meanwhile, MHT adds hormones to a woman's system that is otherwise experiencing diminishing levels and is not used to prevent pregnancy. Many menopause specialists describe MHT as a way to cushion the blow of the loss of hormones as we age.

If you are in perimenopause but don't need to worry about pregnancy (maybe you don't have a male sexual partner or he has gotten a vasectomy), but you are experiencing symptoms, you may want to consider an MHT regimen instead of a hormonal birth control method depending on your bleeding profile and very individualized medical risk factors (such as a history of smoking or blood clots). As usual, the approach is very nuanced and must be done via shared decision-making between a woman and her provider.

What exactly is MHT?

Menopausal hormone therapy typically refers to prescription estrogen and/or progesterone (the other well-known hormone, testosterone, will be discussed further in Chapter 10). MHT can be prescribed in various forms, combinations, and treatment plans. These days we have many prescription options for what is known as "bioidentical hormone therapy," which means the medications have the same molecular structure of the hormones our bodies make. Such drugs are often marketed as more natural, but they are not necessarily safer than traditional MHT synthetic hormones, including conjugated equine estrogens (derived from pregnant horse urine). Sometimes women say they want to avoid "synthetic" medications, but in reality, all drugs made in a lab are synthetic. Menopause experts like Drs. Sharon Malone and Mary Claire Haver generally encourage women to try not to worry too much about marketing labels.[55]

The FDA has approved many hormone therapy options in standardized forms and dosages, but sometimes women need customized versions of medication that they get from compounding pharmacies based on their clinical provider's prescription. Per professional organizations like ACOG and The American Society for Reproductive Medicine (ASRM), compounded MHT is not necessarily bad, as it can help meet a woman's specific needs (e.g., a woman with a peanut allergy may need a compounded form of progesterone that eliminates peanut oil); but FDA-approved formulations are preferred, since they are more studied and better regulated.[56] You should be advised of all options depending on your personal circumstances.

For most women, FDA-approved bioidentical forms of estrogen and progesterone are used as a first-line treatment option and are often covered by insurance plans—though coverage varies widely. If you do need a compounded version of the medication, it is unlikely that your insurance will cover it. You may also prefer a certain method (like a gel) but have to first try another method (like a patch) before the desired method is covered. If this sounds unnecessary and painful—both physically and mentally—to you, that's because it is. But, we're women, so we're expected to add this BS to our to-do lists.

How is MHT administered?

MHT can be systemic (which means that it is medicine introduced to the bloodstream and can impact the whole body, affecting mood, cardiovascular health, and/or symptoms like hot flashes or joint pain) or local (meaning it affects only the spot at which it is applied and does not go into the bloodstream in appreciable amounts). Women can use either or both forms depending on their needs and preferences. In general, as MHT, estrogen and progesterone can be prescribed and consumed in the following ways.

Estrogen can be taken in the form of:

- **Pills ingested by mouth.**
  This is a good option for women who want to be able to easily adjust dosage with their provider as needed but may not be ideal for women with a history of blood clot issues (for whom transdermal options—via the skin—are preferred) or who have trouble remembering daily medication.

- **A patch that's like a sticker that usually goes on the lower stomach or upper butt area.**

  This is typically changed once or twice a week and can also be easily adjusted in terms of dosage, but the adhesive may cause skin irritation. I've also been told that the patch may not be as effective for women who engage in frequent swimming or hot yoga or sauna use.

- **A gel or spray.**

  These topical options are usually applied on the arm or inner thigh (each brand will give instructions in its packaging). Women often start with one press or pump and may increase as needed. Sometimes getting the right dosage can take some trial and error. A few minutes for the medication to dry are required before getting dressed or engaging in physical contact with others, while a few hours are required before bathing.

- **A ring inserted into the vagina.**

  There are both local and systemic vaginal ring options (the former helps alleviate vaginal dryness and other genitourinary discomfort, while the latter can also help with additional symptoms like hot flashes, since the entire body absorbs estrogen). A ring has to be replaced about every 90 days and can be done without a medical provider's help, but that may take some practice (if you're used to a birth control ring, it's a similar insertion process).

- **Vaginal creams or tablets.**

  These are localized to the vagina and not systemic, and so are generally considered safe for all women (even those with estrogen-receptive breast cancer histories, which is discussed further

below). Some women find the cream messy, but most are very appreciative of the relief it provides from genitourinary pain. Women can use vaginal cream or tablets (which basically melt after being inserted into the vaginal canal via an applicator) in addition to other forms of MHT, as medically indicated.

If a woman is being prescribed systemic estrogen and still has a uterus, she *must* also be prescribed something that protects her uterus, typically a progesterone. This is because estrogen alone can stimulate the lining of the uterus and cause endometrial hyperplasia, which can lead to a type of uterine cancer.

Progesterone can be taken in the form of:

- **Pills ingested by mouth.**
  The form of bioidentical progesterone that providers will prescribe is known as oral micronized progesterone, for which the dosage and frequency will vary for each woman. It can be taken every day ("continuously") or at certain dosages during certain times each month ("cyclically"). Bioidentical micronized progesterone is believed to not cause breast cancer (and is different from the synthetic version used in the WHI study). It's generally not absorbed well through the skin, so that is why the pill method is used. The oral version's side effects can include drowsiness or breast tenderness.

- **Pills inserted into the vagina.**
  Sometimes this off-label route is suggested for women who are sensitive to the side effects from the oral version, though it's the same capsule, just inserted into the body in different ways. Practi-

tioners will usually have their patients insert the pill vaginally at night before bedtime.

- **Intrauterine device.**
  Progestin-releasing IUDs provide contraception, help alleviate erratic and heavy bleeding, and protect the endometrial lining sufficiently (even if estrogen is also taken).

Some women, especially those in early perimenopause, may benefit from a course of progesterone only. Some women do well with some estrogen at certain points in their cycle rather than continuously. There are now new drug options that provide a combination of estrogen *and* an estrogen-antagonist (also known as a selective estrogen receptor modulator or SERM), which acts like a progesterone by protecting the uterine lining but may be better for women who don't react well to progesterone.

See, MHT is *incredibly* individualized!

Once women have experienced menopause, their needs change less frequently, so treatment can be more straightforward. But perimenopause symptoms change as women change and should continuously be reevaluated with one's healthcare provider. Dr. Mandelberger summarized, "There are going to be highs and lows. Those fluctuations in hormones may trigger new or different levels of symptoms, so we may have to adjust hormone therapy in response." Dr. Robbins also acknowledged that hormone therapy during perimenopause requires frequent tweaking: "Perimenopause treatment is complex, usually more complex than postmenopause."

Accordingly, she encourages frequent check-ins between patients and providers once a treatment plan has been established. "At a minimum, I think a woman who is being treated for menopause symptoms should be seen every three to six months. I tend to check in more frequently with my patients, especially if they are on a hormone therapy regimen. I think it's really important to see how it's going based on how a woman reports she is feeling." Dr. Hertel likewise said, "Every time we make a change to their regimen, I see women as needed, or every two to three months or so until they are feeling good." She reiterated, "Perimenopause means that hormones and symptoms are fluctuating. So a hormone therapy approach that may have worked well for a while can change. And that's OK, we'll get through it together."

What are the potential side effects of hormone therapy?

The former lawyer in me wants to take the opportunity to remind you (again!) this is all general information, and *not* individualized medical advice. Please keep in mind that hormone therapy is now determined to be generally "safe and beneficial," according to many experts.[57] As with *any* medical treatment, though, there are indeed potential side effects or risks to hormone therapy. Let's start with potential side effects, which may be felt more potently upon beginning MHT and should be raised with your healthcare provider to see if modifications are warranted. As mentioned above, estrogen alone for a woman with a uterus is not recommended due to its potential effects on the uterine lining that can lead to endometrial cancer, a kind of uterine cancer that starts in the uterus's lining. Progesterone, meanwhile, can cause a sedative feeling (so many women take it before bed because of its relaxing effects) or water retention (think of the bloating feeling before a period; that is due to your rising levels of progesterone).

For the common treatment combo of transdermal estrogen and oral progesterone, one of the most common side effects is abnormal or unscheduled bleeding. Such bleeding, warned Dr. Mandelberger, "is not necessarily benign, so if it happens, you must tell your healthcare provider to rule out other causes like a uterine polyp or endometrial hyperplasia (also known as uterine pre-cancer)." Note: Please tell everyone you know that bleeding *post*menopause must be raised with your provider, as it is a top warning sign of endometrial cancer, the most common gynecological cancer, yet a 2024 study revealed that more than one-third of women do not recognize such bleeding as a key symptom.[58]

Other side effects of MHT can include some old familiar friends: tender breasts, mood changes, acne, headaches, difficulty sleeping, dizziness, or increased anxiety. "Some of the issues we are trying to treat can be worsened with hormone therapy, though that is pretty rare," Dr. Mandelberger described. "That's why we play around with the treatment options until we get it right for the symptoms the patient is experiencing at that time, which usually takes a few months." And sometimes side effects can be offset by other treatments; Dr. Robbins shared that some of the side effects of testosterone, for example, can include acne or hair shedding/loss, "but those can often be counteracted with topical or oral medications, if appropriate for the patient."

How do I know if I shouldn't take MHT?

Please speak with a qualified medical provider, ideally one who is specifically trained in menopause care and up-to-date on current guidelines, to make a determination as to whether you are truly not a candidate for menopausal hormone therapy. Many women I know assume they should avoid it because they've had health issues like certain cancers. But research continues to evolve and clarify such assumptions. In 2024, for example, a study was released suggesting that systemic hormone therapy does *not* increase cancer-specific mortality in women with various cancer types, including common cancers like lung, colorectal, and melanoma (but, excluding breast cancer, which we'll discuss more in a moment).[59]

For now, menopausal hormone therapy is generally (though not absolutely or always) contraindicated (meaning, not recommended) for women with:

- Heart health issues including known coronary heart disease or cardiovascular risk factors, conditions like venous thromboembolism and pulmonary embolism, a history of stroke, or congenital heart disease;
- Active, acute liver disease;
- Unexplained vaginal bleeding; or
- Active estrogen-sensitive cancer, including breast or uterine/endometrial cancer.[60]

Keep in mind, there are (as usual) nuances, and every situation is unique. For example, The Menopause Society has issued guidelines that even though "hormone therapy is generally contraindicated in women with estrogen-responsive cancers, hormone therapy may be used to treat bothersome menopause symptoms in women with low-grade, Stage I endometrial cancer after hysterectomy."[61] So please do not assume you can't take MHT without comprehensive conversations based on the latest available information, especially if you are suffering from your symptoms.

What if I don't want to take MHT?

Menopause can be thought of as a natural phase of life—and some women view this as indicating that no medical intervention is needed. However, one could argue that getting ill is also natural, and many women would choose to treat an illness with medicine if it's making them feel bad. Similarly, menopause symptoms can potentially be treated with medication like menopausal hormone therapy. *Suffering through menopause is not necessary.*

Of course, though, if you don't want to take MHT, you don't have to! Maybe your symptoms don't bother you or maybe you want to explore other options—and that's fine. "Women should have agency and autonomy over their bodies and healthcare," agreed Kathy Casey, a doctor of acupuncture and Chinese medicine and the Clinic Director of Touchstone Acupuncture in Westchester County, New York. Dr. Casey has had success helping menopausal women's quality of life through an acupuncture course of about 12 weeks. "We nudge the body to do what it does best, to release biochemicals and regulate the nervous systems. We honor the person that is in the body, giving them encouragement, optimism, and hope that their body was created to go through menopause." She provides hypno-acupuncture treatments to help women release emotional blocks, manage uncomfortable symptoms, and integrate various conscious and subconscious factors to achieve meaningful and sustainable change.

In addition to acupuncture and hypnosis, other mind/body interventions for menopause symptoms can include guided imagery and other forms of biofeedback and relaxation techniques, aromatherapy, reflexology, and time-limited and action-oriented CBT to modify cognitive interpretations and behavior choices.[62] Cognitive behavioral therapy can be particularly helpful for vasomotor, stress, sleep, and mood symptoms.[63] We'll discuss it in further detail in Chapter 8 and explore other options, like potentially helpful lifestyle changes, in Chapter 9.

Nonhormonal medications may also be helpful to treat symptoms. Dr. Messer explained, "For patients who are not candidates for or who choose not to pursue menopausal hormone therapy, we still have a few tricks up our sleeves, including the use of Veozah (or fezolinetant) and Relizen (a pollen extract supplement) for hot flashes, Revaree or other hormone-free, hyaluronic-based vaginal inserts for vaginal dryness, SSRIs for insomnia and mood changes, etc." Over the last couple of years, guidance has been released regarding new nonhormone options that treat vasomotor symptoms by targeting certain neurons of the hypothalamus; experts expect more scientific advances to come.[64]

If I do decide to use MHT, do I have to worry about risks to my heart health?

The 2002 WHI study indicated that hormone therapy could (note: not *would*) lead to a small increased risk of heart health outcomes including heart disease, stroke, and blood clots. But please (!) recall that there were many flaws in the way that study was interpreted, especially since it focused only on postmenopausal women who had experienced menopause years prior (the women in the study ranged in age from 50 to 79, with the average age of 63). So, applying its results to younger women who are in perimenopause would not be accurate.

"For older women who start hormone therapy later on, including postmenopause, there *may* be increased risk of blood clots, pulmonary embolism, stroke, or cardiovascular disease if preexisting," acknowledged Dr. Mandelberger. "But that data should not be extrapolated to younger women who are starting hormone treatment in perimenopause." Additionally, the estrogen used in the WHI study was taken orally by pill; as menopause expert Dr. Lauren Streicher explained to *NPR* in 2024: "A better option for people at risk of clots is to take estrogen through the skin, via a patch, a cream, or gel."[65]

Furthermore, in the years since the 2002 WHI study, research has revealed that hormone therapy is safe for heart health of the average woman under 60, including postmenopausal women.[66] In 2019, the American College of Cardiology suggested that women who have a less than 5 percent risk factor according to their ASCVD (Atherosclerotic Cardiovascular Disease Risk Assessment) score, which they would evaluate with a cardiologist, are generally acceptable candidates for menopausal hormone therapy.[67] In 2020, the American Heart Association asserted: "The evidence supports cardiovascular benefit for MHT initiated early among women with premature or surgical menopause and within 10 years of menopause in women with natural menopause. The benefits of MHT (i.e., including lower rates of diabetes, reduced insulin resistance, and protection from bone loss) appear to outweigh risks for the majority of early menopausal women."[68] This is really important, because heart disease is the number one cause of death for women in the United States.[69]

In sum, when it comes to heart health, NYU cardiologist Anais Hausvater explained that if women are suffering through menopause symptoms and want to use menopausal hormone therapy to alleviate them, they should explore it as an option. "There are even some studies that show lower risk of cardiovascular disease with MHT when initiated early." She told me she encourages all women, including those with higher risk due to a history of blood clotting or congenital issues or other risk factors, to discuss the risks and benefits of hormone therapy with their healthcare provider. If they do pursue MHT, women should continue to undergo blood pressure screening and monitoring (which may be particularly important for those who engage in estrogen-only MHT).[70]

Will MHT cause breast cancer?

This is one of the most common concerns about hormone therapy risk that I hear among women of my generation, an echo from our mothers' generation.

"Estrogen via menopausal hormone therapy does *not cause* breast cancer," according to Dr. Hertel. It could, however, feed off estrogen receptor-positive cancerous cells already present in the body.[71] "This is partly why screening and early detection measures like mammograms are so important," Dr. Hertel emphasized. In the meantime, "Undoing the damage of the 2002 WHI study is going to be a *long* process," reflected Shieva Ghofrany, MD, the OB/GYN whose personal experiences with fertility issues and gynecologic cancer contribute to her passion for helping women utilize an integrative, empowering approach to their own healthcare.

"It's been more than 20 years, and I still have to dispel the myth that estrogen causes breast cancer on a daily basis," described Givargidze. "That claim from the 2002 WHI study has been refuted. Actually, in the WHI we saw that women who took only estrogen (because the uterus had been removed via hysterectomy) had a lower risk of developing breast cancer!" Dr. Robbins further elucidated: "Estrogen never actually showed an increased risk of breast cancer but rather—for the women who had gotten hysterectomies and didn't need progesterone to protect the uterus—about 20 percent reduction in risk when taken as estrogen-only hormone therapy." As experts often point out, if estrogen caused breast cancer, we would expect rates of breast cancer to decline after menopause, when estrogen levels are naturally lower—but instead, they rise (even for women not using hormone therapy). Interpreting the WHI study's data to say that hormone therapy causes breast cancer has been called a "misleading conclusion"[72] and "one of the biggest screw-ups in modern medicine"[73] by various prominent medical experts.

As with all medications, though, there may be a risk depending on your own body and medical issues. For women with uteruses who do need the combination of estrogen and progesterone to lower their risk of developing endometrial cancer, research shows there may be a very slight increased risk of breast cancer. But the medical field continues to evolve, and experts are trying to educate women on what the risks actually mean. In 2024, Dr. JoAnn Manson (the WHI investigator we heard from in Chapter 3) told *The Washington Post*: "'Putting the risk into perspective, it's the equivalent of the excess risk of breast cancer associated with drinking one to two alcoholic beverages daily … The absolute risk is low, and all choices involve trade-offs.'"[74] Such a perspective was repeated at The Menopause Society's 2024 annual meeting among the world's leading menopause experts.

What about MHT and women who have family histories of breast or other cancers?

I was pleasantly surprised to learn from several of the experts I spoke with that there is no family cancer history, including a family history of breast cancer, that would automatically rule out the use of hormone therapy to treat menopause symptoms. "A family history of breast or any cancer is *not* an absolute contraindication of hormone therapy," Dr. Robbins confirmed. "A family history does *not* increase your baseline risk of breast cancer upon taking hormones."

Rather, a family history can be thought of as a clue that prompts discussion and reflection and potential additional procedures to gather knowledge so a patient can fully understand her risks. The providers I spoke with encourage all patients be up-to-date with health screenings, the general guidelines for which are discussed further in Chapter 14. Regular self-breast exams are also recommended, because you know your body (and any changes to it) best.

Genetic testing may be worth pursuing as well, as it can have a profound impact on how one chooses to navigate their health and the menopause transition. Kyle Koeppel Mann, my friend since preschool, is one woman whose genetics have played a huge role in her healthcare. Kyle is a lawyer and writer who advocates for women to share their stories to encourage prevention where possible; her mommy, my mom's friend Sherri, died in 1992 when Kyle was seven, three months after being diagnosed with colon cancer and at the young age of 38. When Kyle was 19 years old, she was diagnosed with Lynch syndrome, a genetic mutation that causes numerous kinds of cancers, including colon, stomach, pancreatic, ovarian, uterine, and cervical.

Given her condition and her family history, Kyle long planned to have her uterus and ovaries removed after bearing children so that she would not have to continue with regular painful endometrial biopsies and other stressful screenings. She ultimately had emergency surgery immediately after her second son was born due to placenta accreta and increta (where the placenta grew into her uterine wall and could not be removed without risking her life). "I don't make light of the emergency, but I was overjoyed to wake up and realize that I no longer had to worry about planning for a hysterectomy and oophorectomy," Kyle shared.

Her joy came alongside surgically induced menopause at age 34. "I'd had concerns about feeling feminine when my uterus, ovaries, cervix, and fallopian tubes were removed, but the main emotion I felt was relief," Kyle reflected. "The risk reduction for me was worth it." Because she was simultaneously postpartum following the removal of these organs, it was hard for her to assess her hormone changes' effect on her body. For one reason or another, she recalled, "there were a lot of sweaty nights." Now she works with an expert, the aforementioned reproductive endocrinologist Dr. Alexis Melnick, to regulate her symptoms through hormone therapy. "I'm so thankful that I've had the opportunity to engage in trial and error (including different sizes and types of estradiol patches) and find what works for me." Kyle is passionate about educating other women about the potential benefits to MHT even if one has a family cancer history.

The idea that one must work with an open-minded provider who is committed to finding personalized solutions for each patient is a position shared by the top women's healthcare professional organizations. In 2020, The Society of Gynecologic Oncology concluded in a statement endorsed by The Menopause Society (then called NAMS) that the benefits of MHT are likely to outweigh the risks for most people with gynecologic cancer issues like epithelial ovarian cancer (the most common ovarian cancer), early-stage endometrial cancer (the more common and more easily cured uterine cancer), cervical cancer, and people with the BRCA1 or BRCA2 gene mutations or Lynch syndrome.[75]

MHT is still not generally recommended for women with other gynecologic cancers like advanced endometrial cancer or uterine sarcoma (the less common uterine cancer), but menopause experts and women's health advocates still believe that women should be able to make informed choices. This means that they should be provided with all the information relevant to their situation so that they can freely consider the impact of their decisions. "I had a rare type of ovarian cancer," noted Dr. Ghofrany. "When I went through surgical menopause at age 46, I wasn't offered hormone therapy. But now it's been several years, and I have learned more about my personal risks and the potential benefits to my bones and brain. I chose to look at all the data and decided that MHT was appropriate for me."

MHT could be an appropriate option for women with family histories of breast cancer, too. "I often hear, 'I was told I can't take hormone therapy because my mother had breast cancer.' But this kind of blanket statement is false and misleading," clarified Givargidze, the nurse practitioner. "Your choice to take hormone therapy should be based off your individual medical history and the specific risks vs. benefits to you as an individual."

What about women who have had breast cancer themselves?

Age is the biggest risk factor for breast cancer, though breast cancer diagnoses in women under 50 are continuing to rise. This is certainly an important area of health for millennial women. My friend Robyn Grosshandler is one millennial woman with a personal history, which she graciously shares in order to teach and advocate for others. Born in 1985, she had recently become a mother when she got diagnosed with breast cancer that was positive for estrogen and progesterone receptors ("ER/PR+") in 2020, with no family history, and during the early days of the pandemic. "I quickly learned a lot about hormones," she recalled, "because my kind of cancer fed on estrogen and progesterone."'

Upon reviewing her cancer treatment options, Robyn decided to proceed with a double mastectomy (surgery that removes both breasts), take Tamoxifen (a drug that blocks the activity of estrogen in order to stop the growth of tumors), undergo chemotherapy (treatment that destroys cancer cells and prevents tumor growth), and take Lupron (i.e., leuprolide, a hormone therapy injection that is used to treat hormone receptive positive* or "HR+" breast cancer in premenopausal women). "I was told that Lupron makes it so that I don't produce hormones, so it would put me into chemical menopause," Robyn explained. Both Tamoxifen and Lupron can cause menopause symptoms like hot flashes, vaginal discomfort, and mood swings, and because the ovaries are "shut down" with Lupron, medically induced menopause occurs.[76]

"Before my diagnosis, 'menopause' meant nothing to me," Robyn admitted. "The only thing I associated with the term was hot flashes. Then, at just 35, I came to learn what hot flashes were really like." Soon after starting the medications, she started to experience "insane" hot flashes—"dripping sweat incessantly 12 to 15 times a day." Robyn has received injections for Lupron approximately every 12 weeks since 2021 and will continue to do so for the foreseeable future. "Now menopause is part of my daily life."

---

* According to Penn Medicine's Abramson Cancer Center, about two-thirds of breast cancers have at least one type of hormone receptor. See https://www.pennmedicine.org/cancer/types-of-cancer/breast-cancer/types-of-breast-cancer/hormone-positive-breast-cancer.

So what can hormone receptor-positive breast cancer patients or survivors do to alleviate menopause symptoms? "I would not offer menopausal hormone therapy to a woman currently undergoing treatment for breast cancer that involves suppressing the production of hormones," explained Dr. Mandelberger. "If they were to take systemic hormones, that would be directly counteracting their medication. So that is not an option." However, localized hormones, like a vaginal estrogen cream, may still be worth pursuing and are generally considered safe. "It is widely accepted that for breast cancer survivors turned menopausal women with vaginal atrophy, localized estrogen is safe and can be incredibly helpful," confirmed Dr. Melnick, who suggests women collaborate with their oncologists throughout menopause treatment to get individualized care.

These women are not doomed to suffer. As aforementioned, there are nonhormonal treatment options to get some relief. "Many tools are available to relieve menopausal hormone symptoms, even for women who are not candidates for MHT," confirmed Givargidze. "Hypnotherapy, CBT, and targeted pharmaceuticals—meaning medications to target each symptom—have been shown to be effective." Robyn, who receives all her care at Memorial Sloan Kettering Cancer Center in New York (until recently, her medications were prescribed by her oncologist but are now managed by a psychiatrist who specializes in cancer) has tried a variety of strategies to alleviate the impact of her hot flashes. She carries a portable fan and has tried SSRIs. She recently found out about an experimental drug meant to help middle-aged women with bladder control, but that has helped her hot flashes become both less frequent and less severe.

Alison Schram, MD, the gynecologic medical oncologist, explained, "In a patient with a history of a hormonally driven cancer I prefer nonhormonal alternatives for symptomatic menopause—but the individual, specific risks of hormone therapy for each woman must always be weighed against the benefits they may gain based on their personal needs. I have most commonly prescribed SSRIs for menopause-associated hot flashes. Recently, the NK3 receptor antagonist, fezolinetant, was FDA approved and fortunately our armamentarium has expanded."

Ultimately, though, if nonhormonal options are not working to alleviate severe menopause symptoms and she is suffering from poor quality of life, a woman who has had hormone receptive breast cancer may still choose to pursue menopausal hormone therapy. "If the woman is miserable from menopause symptoms, she deserves a nuanced conversation about all of her options with an educated healthcare provider," Dr. Hertel offered, echoing The Menopause Society's 2022 guidance.[77] "Understandably, women with a personal history of breast cancer may not want to go on any kind of hormone therapy because they are scared or want to decrease every risk possible. But they should still be made aware of all of the options." And the options may continue to expand. As proffered in a 2024 study on breast cancer survivors' endocrine consequences: "An absolute ban on MHT for breast cancer survivors does seem incongruous given that pregnancy [during which estrogen levels rise] is not absolutely discouraged."[78] Individualized assessments and shared decision-making are always good ideas.

Is there more information on MHT's potential protective and preventative impacts?

Yes, though we need more.

"Menopausal hormone therapy is not currently recommended as a preventative measure," explained Dr. Melnick. This means that "women who have no menopause symptoms should not take hormone therapy *solely* to prevent future cardiovascular risks," for example, according to Dr. Hausvater, the cardiologist. But, there is a "large and growing body of evidence that shows a cardioprotective effect of estrogens when started in early menopause," Dr. Mandelberger pointed out.[79]

And helping heart health can lead to other benefits, like brain health and overall well-being. Several studies purport that there may be many benefits to using MHT during perimenopause, a time that's often referred to as a window of opportunity to target cardiovascular and neurological risk factors.[80] A 2024 study of nearly 118,000 women in the United Kingdom found that postmenopausal women who had received hormone therapy beginning at approximately age 48 were biologically younger* than those who did not, regardless of socioeconomic background, demonstrating an association between hormone therapy and healthy aging.[81]

---

* Biological age reflects one's health span. It is based on the functioning of various biomarkers, influenced by genetics, nutrition, lifestyle, and other factors, compared with one's chronological age, which is based on when in the calendar you were born. Learn more: Susan Breshnahan, "You Have Two Ages, Chronological and Biological. Here's Why It Matters," *CNN*, updated November 30, 2018, https://www.cnn.com/2018/11/30/health/live-longer-biological-age-intl/index.html.

And while focusing on breast cancer risk is of course incredibly important, we may be worried about the wrong thing. For example, the risk of dying from heart disease is greater than from breast cancer itself for many breast cancer survivors.[82] Perhaps women should be equally if not more concerned about an osteoporotic fracture, which happens more frequently than breast cancers and cardiovascular disease events combined in nearly all race/ethnic groups (except Black women, for whom the number of fractures is similar to the number of CVD events).[83] Fractures may be not only physically painful but also emotionally distressing. They can disrupt one's ability to live independently, which can have serious impacts. They are also quite costly for the individual experiencing them and the healthcare system in general. Estrogen, essentially regarded as an enemy to women's heath since the WHI study, has been shown to decrease fracture risk and prevent or manage osteoporosis.[84]

OK, so in the span of 20-ish years, we've gone from fearing hormone therapy to considering how helpful it might be to prevent lots of scary health issues. What's a girl to do?

It's impossible for me to give an answer about whether to—or when to—start MHT. It used to be recommended that MHT be initiated within 10 years of menopause or before 60, but those guidelines are currently being reconsidered and may be expanded.[85] The experts I spoke to generally agree that exactly when to start hormone therapy needs to be better researched.

In the meantime, I want you to know for certain that you are entitled to more information about it. "Even if you have *no* menopause symptoms, it's worth having a conversation about menopausal hormone therapy as you approach midlife," suggested Dr. Melnick. "This is the point of physicians counseling patients—*everything* has risks and benefits that will be personal to each patient. Women deserve to have doctors who are savvy about menopause and can share the data so women can make comprehensive choices for themselves."

It sounds like millennials navigating menopause should have multiple medical options, right?

Right. As articulated by Stephanie Faubion, MD, MBA (who, since 2019, has held the esteemed roles of the director of the Mayo Clinic's Center for Women's Health and the medical director of The Menopause Society) in 2023 for *The New York Times Magazine*: "'[T]here are very few women who have absolute contraindications [for hormone therapy]… For everyone else[,] the decision [to use it] has to do with the severity of symptoms as well as personal preferences and level of risk tolerance [for women who may have cardiovascular health issues or a personal history of breast cancer, recurrence of which potentially could be affected by MHT].'"[86]

"All risk factors should be taken into account in conversations about options with the patient," explained Dr. Mandelberger of her approach to individualized care. "This is where the art and science of medicine overlap. Every woman is different and as long as she is competent, rational, and well-informed, I believe it should be up to her to balance her highly individualized risk vs. reward of treatment options."

For example, she shared, she recently treated a patient who chose to pursue hormone therapy for menopause symptoms after successfully treating ER+ breast cancer 15 years ago. The patient had been suffering. She was experiencing frequent hot flashes and night sweats, causing her to wake up repeatedly throughout the night, which exacerbated other physical and mental symptoms including mood. This patient confirmed, "I know and understand the data that points to a very small risk of recurrence or newfound breast cancer, and I'm choosing to prioritize my quality of life."

My friend Robyn, too, felt empowered by her ability to make choices regarding her treatments. "At some point I'll have to decide if I want to remove my ovaries, uterus, and cervix. I've been told that potential benefits of doing so would include avoiding the risk of getting cancer in those organs. But, I could risk having my menopause symptoms triple, and I'm currently of the mindset that I'm not ready for that," she reflected. She may still choose to avoid MHT at that point even without her female reproductive organs because of the risk of the estrogen-receptive disease having metastasized somewhere in her body, but that is an assessment she'll consider and make another day.

"For now, I'm avoiding recurrence and minimizing my medications' side effects," Robyn said. "I'm very much focused on keeping my body as healthy as I can—while enjoying living my life." She celebrates her anniversary of being cancer-free every year with a party where guests are encouraged to wear pink, donate to cancer research, and not sweat the small stuff. I'm so proud to be her friend.

HOW CAN MILLENNIALS PREPARE?

Know Your Body, Know Yourself

First, know your body. Know what's "normal" for you—for your cycle, for your mood, for your sleep, for your baseline without any aches and pains—and know that it may not be what others are experiencing. Then, if you feel like something has changed or become "abnormal," get help.

"Not all women experience menopause symptoms," Dr. Mandelberger reiterated. "But if you do, and if that symptom is interfering with your ability to live a fulfilling, healthy life, it's a problem. It could be a common symptom, but one worth treating nonetheless." She urged: "You do not have to ride a wave of pain or discomfort."

"Women should not feel the need to 'white knuckle' it through the early years of menopause," Dr. Messer agreed. That means you do *not* need to accept your inability to remember things, your debilitating joint pain, your struggle to fall back asleep after waking up in the middle of the night, or any other symptoms just because you are getting older. If your quality of life is impaired—or if you just want to feel like yourself again—help is available. "Even though menopause may sound far away, the earlier you can recognize symptoms of perimenopause, the sooner you can address them," asserted Dr. Robbins. "The perimenopause phase can be years-long, but you definitely don't have to be miserable that whole time!"

And hopefully you now understand that medical treatment of menopause symptoms must be tailored to you. You may ultimately choose to pursue hormone therapy (in collaboration with an appropriate provider, of course) based on your symptoms and health history, or you may prefer nonhormonal alternatives, or perhaps you will decide to avoid treatment altogether. You do you, babe. Your body, your choice!

Know How to Access Quality Care

As a culture, we're still dealing with the impact of the incorrect messaging following the 2002 WHI study. I know that even a reference to breast cancer or blood clotting can sound alarming. But I hope you now understand that while hormone therapy has potential risks and benefits (like nearly everything in medicine), it is certainly not unequivocally dangerous for all women. It's not an option you must fear, but rather, an option to learn more about.

I'll give a disclaimer one more time here: I am not a doctor, the doctors I've featured are not *your* doctors, and it is imperative you receive individualized healthcare as you approach and go through menopause.

With that said, how can you access such important, individualized care? I acknowledge that not everyone lives near me or most of the providers I've mentioned in the New York City area. And I understand that concierge medical care, which is amazing for its comprehensiveness, can be costly. Fortunately, quality menopause care is becoming increasingly accessible because of telemedicine and new companies whose mission is to fill this gap in care. Here are some options* that may be available to you, whether you live in Stars Hollow, Laguna Beach, or anywhere in between:

- **Alloy**

  Cofounded by Anne Fulenwider, who inspired my investigation into menopause that ultimately led to this book, Alloy is a telemedicine practice serving patients in the United States (excluding US territories). It also offers free resources on its website, myalloy.com. Alloy patients complete detailed medical intake forms and have the opportunity to share additional information with a doctor who reviews them and then, if appropriate, recommends products that may be prescription or over-the-counter to treat symptoms. "We insist on evidence-based solutions," per Fulenwider, "and we tell it like it is, which our users appreciate." Patients have access to a messaging system in which they can ask questions and follow up with an experienced medical provider. While Alloy does not accept insurance, patients may be eligible for reimbursement depending on their insurance plans or to use HSA or FSA to pay for their products.

- **Elektra**

  Elektra Health provides clinical care from board-certified providers and a digital support and community platform for midlife women, starting with menopause and extending into Medicare years. Elektra is designed to provide virtual care and support—all covered by insurance—for those navigating menopause and in their postmenopausal decades. Elektra's

---

* Information is accurate as of January 2025; please visit each company's website for current offerings and payment options.

patients range in age from 40 to 70. Services include telemedicine care in all 50 states, access to their MD-trained menopause guides or "menopause doulas" (former birth doulas who now specialize in menopause), a supportive community with members-only events, and unlimited chat and support. Patients can book visits with board-certified menopause experts via elektrahealth.com. Elektra is in-network with Medicare and Medicaid, which means Elektra's serving a wide swath of women from a diverse array of socioeconomic backgrounds. It is also HSA/FSA-eligible.

- **Health by Heather Hirsch MD Collaborative**
  Dr. Hirsch, who has been mentioned in previous chapters for her educational media platforms, has trained a team of healthcare providers collectively licensed in nearly all 50 states to provide science-backed advice on menopause and perimenopause through telehealth and in-person in New York visits. Through its website, heatherhirschmd.com/collaborative, women can easily schedule new patient visits with a provider licensed in their state, after which they will have access to a comprehensive intake form, Dr. Hirsch's course covering perimenopause and menopause, and a private Facebook community group frequently visited by the Collaborative providers. They work with a patient's primary healthcare team or gynecologist as needed and, if indicated, will prescribe FDA-approved hormone therapy that can be sent to a local pharmacy. The medications may be covered by insurance, but the Collaborative does not accept insurance for visits; however, patients may be eligible for reimbursement depending on their plans or may be able to use HSA or FSA funds if applicable.

- **Midi**

    A virtual platform that describes itself as a "care company, not a pharmaceutical company" dedicated to "long-term partnership" with patients, Midi offers specialized treatments for common symptoms of perimenopause and postmenopause, including weight and body changes, hot flashes, trouble sleeping, period problems, and more when patients book a visit. Women from all 50 states can sign up at joinmidi.com for the virtual care clinic, whose providers are menopause specialists. Patients fill out user-friendly and detailed forms based on their experiences, meet via secure videoconference with their Midi clinician to discuss their health in-depth, get blood work or imaging to personalize their treatment at local facilities if needed, and collaborate with their providers on treatment options based on their symptoms, unique medical histories, and personal approaches to health. Visits and noncustomized prescriptions are covered by major insurance providers.

These platforms provide not only access to qualified menopause specialists (including those who serve on their boards) but also free educational tools like newsletters and recordings of their expert talks. Definitely utilize (and share) science-backed resources like these!

Know You May Have Options Beyond Western Medicine

While medication is not for every woman, whether or not they have a potential contraindication, every woman should know that medical options exist. A 2024 online study of 223 women aged 28 to 43 revealed that the majority answered "maybe" (60.4 percent) or "yes" (32.3 percent) if they would consider using hormone therapy; yet only 12.1 percent felt well-informed about menopause in general.[87] We must keep learning and sharing information on treatment options!

And treatment options may not include traditional (or Western) medicine altogether. Dr. Casey highlighted other potentially helpful tools like "moxibustion (dried herbs), herbal formulations specific to each unique woman, qigong (movement with breathwork), food considerations in accordance with each woman's constitution (akin to Ayurvedic medicine), and the guiding principal of body-mind-spirit unity." Researchers are currently looking into additional options, like how cannabis and CBD might help provide symptom relief, for example (TLDR: We don't have enough data yet to confirm they are effective treatments, but women often report symptom relief with use of such products).[88]

Many of the menopause experts I spoke with acknowledged that women often like to use dietary supplements like black cohosh or primrose to alleviate symptoms like hot flashes or night sweats, but they tend to be untested and unregulated, so additional research on their efficacy is desired. For now, some medical providers believe in such supplements' placebo effect, as do I—as long as a supplement is safe (doing no harm), its cost is viable, and it's working for you, I believe you should do what you believe is best for you. But, *please* do talk to your healthcare provider and inform them of your preferences so they can inform you of any risks.

And do keep in mind that you can change your mind about treatment options at any time. "You'll get frustrated if you think it's one and done in terms of treatment options," advised Dr. Ghofrany. "Your symptoms will change, medicine evolves, your knowledge will grow as will your providers'. It's most important to know yourself and communicate with your providers."

We now know that the way we treat menopause symptoms is going to be a very personal journey. And personally, I am thrilled to see the rise of accessible resources and treatment options. As we'll learn in the next chapter, we still have a long way to go.

Chapter 7

WOMEN'S HEALTHCARE IN AMERICAN CULTURE

So, OK, you're probably going, *Does anyone actually care about women's healthcare, or what?*

I don't want to be a downer, but seriously, it too often feels like issues that primarily impact women (particularly those related to their reproductive health) are simply not valued in American culture.

Let me prove this point by starting with a look at the unfair prices we have to pay for products and services we as women *need* for our health.

Did you know that personal care products marketed toward women are usually more expensive than those geared toward men, even if they have nearly identical ingredients? For example, in 2015, the New York City Department of Consumer Affairs engaged in a study of national retailers and found 42 percent of the time, women are charged an average of 7 percent more than men for "what is ostensibly the same product,"[89] including toys, accessories, clothing across all age groups, personal care products, or senior/home healthcare products. As noted by the researchers, "In the aggregate, over the course of a female consumer's lifetime, these discrepancies would have a much larger financial impact, given that, on average, personal care products cost 13 percent more for women than men."[90]

This gendered phenomenon is often referred to as "the pink tax" and feels particularly unjust given that women in this country are still subject to a stark gender pay gap and as such, not making as much money as their male counterparts.[91] As of 2024, women in the United States are paid 78 cents for every dollar paid to men, with the pay gap widest for women of color. Accordingly, women employed in the US "lose a combined total of more than $1.6 trillion every year due to the wage gap."[92] Moreover, mothers tend to experience a penalty in which they make, on average, 63 cents for every dollar paid to fathers.[93]

If you look like the angry red emoji with the expletive box right now, I understand. In fact, let's take a cue from Alloy's Fulenwider and all just say it together ... What the fuck?!

I'll add some fuel to the fire that I hope you use to help me burn down the patriarchy. Let's get back to periods; this is a book about menopause, after all. People with male reproductive systems have no use for period products (also commonly referred to as feminine hygiene products, a phrase I don't really care for, since I think it connotes a lack of cleanliness during menstruation)—but women do need them, of course. And, as long as you are premenopause, their cost adds up.

For example, reports have shown that "[t]he average woman [in the US] will use about 240 tampons a year, which comes out to about $50 each year with tax," as consumers still have to pay a sales tax on them in multiple states,* despite their being essential.[94] Let's not forget the potential costs of items like panty liners, overnight pads, new underwear due to stains, pain relief medication, and other products that may be used in addition to those expensive tampons.[95] Put another way, if the average woman in the US spends "about $20 on feminine hygiene products per cycle, [that adds] up to about $18,000 over her lifetime,"[96] a cost that males do not even need to consider. And the costs seem to be going up due to inflation; a recent report showed that the average price of a pack of sanitary pads rose 41 percent between 2019 and 2024, while tampons' average price increased by 36 percent.[97]

This is ultimately a lot of money, especially for low-income women, and can be prohibitive or even dangerous. A 2023 study of teenagers and adults who menstruate reflected that nearly one in four teens have struggled to afford period products in the US (suffering from "period poverty"), while 40 percent of teens and 52 percent of adults

---

* As of November 2024, 21 states still tax period products as "nonessential goods" (though products like Rogaine [for men's hair loss] and Viagra [you already know this one!] are considered medical necessities; learn more and get reimbursed by a wonderful coalition of women's health product companies at www.tampontaxback.com.

have worn period products for longer than recommended.[98] In 2024, a study found that it went up to one in three teens and young adults in the US who couldn't afford or access menstrual products, a widespread need affecting young people despite differences in race, ethnicity, neighborhood, or health insurance.[99]

Per the CDC, "[w]earing a pad or period underwear for too long can lead to a rash or an infection,"[100] and that's basically the least of our problems. As noted in a 2023 study about period poverty (dubbed a "neglected public health issue" therein), the "prolonged use of menstrual products, such as pads, tampons, or menstrual cups, increases the risk of infections such as urinary tract infection and bacterial vaginosis."[101] To quote my Cuban Jewish grandmother Helen: *Oy, oy, oy,* this is *no bueno.*

Let's not forget about the toxic shock syndrome[102] risk associated with tampon use. It's been nearly three decades since I got my first period, and every time I go to the bathroom while menstruating I pause to precisely count the hours that have passed since I last changed my tampon. "Tampons left too long inside can kill you! But look at our new cute packaging!" was (and still is) the vibe. When I first started writing this book, I was aware of only one rare but life-threatening concern when it came to tampons' health risks—but that soon changed. In July 2024, researchers published a study finding toxic metals, including arsenic and lead, in more than 12 frequently purchased tampon brands.[103] Cool!

Don't fret, ladies. If you want to avoid getting your period and dealing with the multiple financial, emotional, and potential health-related costs of monthly bleeding, consider a hormonal intrauterine device to help suppress your period. Just keep in mind that an IUD insertion can feel like a series of period cramps or an extremely painful pinch and that you likely have to proactively ask for pain relief because most providers will insist it's quick (maybe, but also, *ow!*).

Seeing red yet? (Pun intended, I can't resist.)

It does feel like women's health isn't properly cared for in our culture, doesn't it? And I haven't even explicitly mentioned the attacks on women's reproductive rights over the past few years. But buckle up, because now I will.

In June 2022, the United States Supreme Court overturned *Roe v. Wade*, the landmark 1973 decision that ruled the federal Constitution protected the right to have an abortion prior to fetal viability as part of a woman's right to privacy. Since then, as of January 2025, 19 states have banned abortion in nearly all circumstances or restrict it to earlier in the pregnancy than the standard set in *Roe* (many states now ban abortion after six weeks of pregnancy, yet often women don't even know they are pregnant at that time due to a history of irregular periods or a lack of education).[104] More states are in the process of enacting legislation to limit it.* Both women and their healthcare providers have been criminalized for accessing or providing abortion-related healthcare.

---

* The Center for Reproductive Rights updates abortion laws by state at https://reproductiverights.org/maps/abortion-laws-by-state.

And let me be clear. Abortion is healthcare.* Women have needlessly died after being denied care. Pregnant women may need or want an abortion for a variety of reasons, including medical issues impacting them or their fetus, or because of the potentially violent or nonconsensual way the fetus was conceived, or because they did not intend to have a child at this time in their lives due to financial or other concerns. It's really none of our business why. If you don't want an abortion, don't have one. That is your choice. And women's ability to make whatever choices they want about their own bodies and health should not be restricted.

As described by the authors of a 2023 cross-sectional study, "access to wanted reproductive healthcare, including contraceptive services and abortion, allows individuals to exercise their bodily autonomy and control if and/or when they want to have children, which can ultimately improve individuals' well-being and quality of life."[105] And yet, here we are. Women's mental health, physical health, safety, and financial security are being impacted because people want to control them—or, at best, don't care enough about them.

It's not just access to reproductive healthcare like abortion that has been limited (though that should be enough to make you really, really mad), but also access to routine reproductive healthcare screenings, birth control (that can, as a reminder, be used not only

---

* Professional organizations like The American College of Obstetricians and Gynecologists agree; See, e.g., https://www.acog.org/advocacy/facts-are-important/abortion-is-healthcare. Entire families and communities can suffer from such restrictions, too: Abortion bans have also been associated with higher rates of infant mortality, especially for populations that already experience higher than average rates; See Alison Gemmill et al., "US Abortion Bans and Infant Mortality," *JAMA* (2025), DOI: 10.1001/jama.2024.28517.

for preventing pregnancy but also for helping manage debilitating cramps, stubborn hormonal acne, and painful perimenopause symptoms), fertility treatments, and more. A July 2024 report confirmed that many states in the US currently lack accessible and affordable reproductive healthcare, with statistics worse for women of color throughout the country. Even comprehensive sex education is under attack by extremists. And sexually transmitted infections and unwanted pregnancies cannot be prevented or properly treated without safe, quality reproductive healthcare.

"We've come so far in so many ways regarding women's health, but now we're going backwards," sadly observed Deborah Duke, the long-term women's health nurse. It's terrifying. Tragically, at the time of my writing this, we have fewer rights than the generation of women before us. I'm worried about what this means for our daughters. And honestly, I'm also worried about what it means for us.

Menopause treatment is part of women's reproductive healthcare. If we want to be able to access the quality healthcare we deserve during menopause, we must advocate for quality healthcare for all women, at all phases of our lives—period.

HOW CAN MILLENNIALS PREPARE?

Recognize the Impact of Better Healthcare Provider Training

Limitations on reproductive healthcare is not the fault of providers. But at least with issues like menopause, it's clear they need more comprehensive training.

Some schools (not enough, but some) do have amazing training programs for OB/GYNs and other healthcare providers. Dr. Lilli Dash Zimmerman, the millennial fertility specialist, completed her Obstetrics and Gynecology residency program at the Hospital of the University of Pennsylvania, under the tutelage of Dr. Ann Steiner, whom she calls a "trailblazer and incredible teacher." Penn Medicine's menopause training program started in 2012. Dr. Steiner said of the need for menopause training in 2017: "'There has been a noticeable lack of education about menopause and what that means for today's woman, both on the patient and provider side… As a patient, understanding what to expect and how to manage it is the key to getting through it as smoothly as possible, and helps them to feel like they're in control of what's going on and not just a victim of aging.'"[106]

Meanwhile, the Center for Sexual Medicine and Menopause at Northwestern Memorial Hospital in Chicago was founded by Dr. Lauren Streicher in 2017 to offer specialized care in menopause and sexual health. She found that these issues were not getting the attention they deserved because of a combination of patient embarrassment and provider (under-)education. Of the Center, she told *CBS News Chicago* in 2017, "'It's not just treating these things [related to menopause], it's doing research. It's educating other doctors and nurses on how to take care of patients that have these issues'"; in 2018, she recounted to *AARP Magazine* that the clinic got "'very busy'" quickly because it filled "'a huge unmet need... Menopause touches every aspect of a woman's overall health.'"[107]

It's been several years since, yet healthcare providers in the United States still do not get adequate training in menopause despite its prevalence as a healthcare issue, which is why so many of the providers mentioned in Chapter 3 and throughout this book have had to seek it out on their own. In 2024, OB/GYN Nanette Santoro offered this perspective on the universality of menopause and the need to care for it: "15% of women will experience infertility, whereas *all of them will experience menopause* provided they do not undergo an untimely death ... [There is] a crying need for more adequately trained menopause practitioners."[108]

Fortunately, physicians, researchers, and students themselves have been increasingly calling for better menopause training, to better care for women.[109] Professional organizations like The Menopause Society and The International Menopause Society have also begun explicitly encouraging healthcare professionals to get better versed in menopause symptoms and treatment management and offer comprehensive, collaborative discussions with their patients.[110]

It's never too late for providers to get more education. And when they do, both they and their patients benefit!

Fertility specialists, for example, can naturally add menopause care to their services given their expertise in the endocrine system and passion for supporting women. Dr. Melnick described: "About 5 to 10 percent of my current practice is treating patients with menopausal hormone therapy. It's a nice mix of work, especially when I can continue to work with patients from fertility issues through the menopause transition." She noted that she was largely self-taught by training she sought out and her mentor, since she didn't learn it in school.

Dr. Rebbecca Hertel (who, as aforementioned, also had to proactively seek out training) currently pays it forward by training medical students because she recognizes the deep need to teach as many colleagues and up-and-coming providers as possible about menopause. Meanwhile, a colleague of mine in the mental health field, psychiatrist Dr. Marra Ackerman, colaunched a fellowship in women's mental health at NYU in order to give medical students experience across a woman's reproductive lifespan, including perimenopause. "There hasn't been a whole lot of information on the menopause transition in reproductive psychiatry training, so I want to educate the next generation of providers and share my experience in managing hormone-related mood issues," she explained.

And providers must continue to learn, or they'll risk doing a disservice to their patients.

As Dr. Alicia Robbins, the OB/GYN and menopause specialist, reflected, "Medicine is constantly evolving in terms of research and data, and healthcare providers must evolve with it. If your practitioner is dismissing your symptoms because of an outdated understanding or an unwillingness to learn, you deserve better."

Vote

At least until the current administration, US schools and policymakers have been slowly but surely addressing the gaps in women's healthcare via education, resources, or otherwise. And they should—not only because it's right to do so but also because it's what the people want.

For example, an August 2024 poll found that about 77 percent of Americans agree that menstrual supplies should be as freely available as toilet paper in public school and university bathrooms.[111] Several states have created policies to provide free access to period products at schools, but we need all to do so.[112] Former teacher and vice presidential candidate Tim Walz, for instance, signed a 2023 education law as governor of Minnesota that included a mandate to provide free menstrual supplies to students in grades 4 through 12.[113] In August 2024, New York governor Kathy Hochul signed into law a bill that my own local assemblymember Amy Paulin authored to address period poverty by requiring public colleges and universities to provide free menstrual products in their restrooms (the issue was brought to Paulin's attention by two local high school students, a pair of sisters named Katherine and Elizabeth Sanchez—you go, girls!).[114]

Such legislation is reflective of the power of constituents who demand change. In other words, it may feel like too few people care about menopause and women's healthcare, but those who do care (like us!) truly can make a difference if and when they advocate for more. Consider the new guidelines around IUD insertion released in August 2024 by the US Centers for Disease Control and Prevention—after years of women complaining that their pain was not being taken seriously, the CDC finally gave updated recommendations for clinicians on informing all patients about potential plain and personalizing pain management plans for each individual patient.[115]

Earlier in 2024, President Joe Biden issued an Executive Order creating a $12 billion fund to expand and improve research on women's health, including women's health at midlife.[116] Among other groundbreaking and much-needed decrees, the order includes directives to government agencies to identify ways to improve menopause-related issues and the clinical care women receive, to develop new resources for menopause symptom prevention and treatment, and to advance research related to the impact of perimenopause and menopause on heart, brain, and bone health. In September 2024, Jill Biden revealed a plan to spend $500 million annually on women's health research to help address inequities.[117] In December 2024, the Biden administration held its first-ever conference on women's health research.

So some people do indeed care about menopause and women's healthcare, hooray!

Of course, we cannot take that for granted, as, well, things in DC and beyond can quickly change. We need our elected officials to continue to actually care about women and their health. We also need more comprehensive and current information; professional organizations like the American Heart Association and The Menopause Society are calling for more research, as are individual professionals. "I would love to see—among many other studies—a randomized controlled trial of transdermal estradiol [the estrogen hormone used in MHT] and progesterone vs. placebo when started early in perimenopause, and follow those patients for years," Dr. Mandelberger, the menopause specialist, reflected. "It would be incredibly informative to learn the impact on risks, heart disease, dementia, breast cancer, and more."

You know who can fund such research? Our government!* "The budget for the National Institutes of Health, the world's largest source of medical research funding, is approved by Congress," explained Dr. Brittany Barreto, the FemTech expert. But despite the fact that women are about half the population, women's health research accounts for only about 10.8 percent of the NIH budget.[118] That must change in order for women's healthcare to change. We must elect people to power who actually prioritize women's health and who will make decisions about funding and policies accordingly.

Advocate (Loudly) on All Levels

We must also call attention to menopause-related legislation and policies that our elected officials are or should be working on. You can learn more about proposed laws related to menopause care from the National Menopause Foundation's Policy Institute. Via Let's Talk Menopause, you can (and should) easily send a message to

---

* It's OK if you needed a little Civics refresher in addition to Biology. You're not the only one!

your member of Congress regarding the Menopause Research & Equity Act of 2023* (a bipartisan bill that would direct the National Institutes of Health to focus investments and conduct long-term research, including on new treatments for menopause symptoms) or to the FDA urging them to remove the outdated misleading "boxed warning" on vaginal estrogen products (which overstates the risk and prevents many women from accessing relief for genitourinary menopause symptoms).

Women continue to be harmed by misinformation and alarmist attitudes reflected in things like the boxed warning, and sharing our experiences helps create change. Otherwise, we will continue to suffer in silence and solitude. I can't keep track of the number of Facebook mom group posts I've seen recently from "Anonymous" describing being dismissed by providers for what are probably perimenopause symptoms or being charged out-of-pocket for menopause-related visits because their in-network providers are saying the longer visits are not covered by their health insurance (if this has happened to you, contact the lawyer Susan Frankel to assess your options!).

Women are basically screaming and crying on the internet, but we need to take our rage to real life. "'What does it take to get us out of this?' The Menopause Society's Dr. Stephanie Faubion pondered in September 2024, of the need to dispel hormone therapy myths and spread accurate information and resources on menopause. "It is going to take women getting angry.'"[119]

---

* H.R.6749—Menopause Research and Equity Act of 2023. Track its progress at Congress.Gov.

If you feel angry that so little care is given to women's healthcare, please know that I care. And menopause is an issue that we care about, together. In addition to supporting the work of Let's Talk Menopause and the National Menopause Foundation, you can help raise awareness about women's reproductive health needs by calling attention to period poverty. The Alliance for Period Supplies is a nonprofit that works throughout the US; check out its list of allied programs[120] to donate to local organizations supporting women and girls in need of menstrual supplies. And even if you don't have resources right now, you have your voice. Normalizing conversations about these issues is a great and important contribution, even if only among your own community.

We have to keep (or start) being loud. We have to keep having conversations about menopause, menstruation, and women's health with each other, with the men in our lives, and with our children. We have to keep teaching, learning, and showing that we care by speaking about these issues. It starts with us.

I'm here if you want to talk.

Chapter 8

MENOPAUSE AND MENTAL HEALTH

• • • • • • • • • • • • • • • • • •

Checking in—how are you doing?

Seriously, how are you feeling?

It can be really overwhelming, I know. I've thrown a lot at you—medical terms, scary symptoms, information on misinformation, fears about cancer and cardiovascular risks, sad stories from women who have already been through it and felt lonely, gender discrimination in multiple layers of American culture, gaps in healthcare training, government inaction, and more… Oh my! And we're barely halfway through the book!

In the last chapter I talked a lot about education and advocacy, two topics that have always been near and dear to my heart. After college, I chose to simultaneously pursue my law and social work degrees back home in New York City. I wanted to learn how to become the best possible advocate for women, and for many years did so as an attorney helping them get orders of protection, visas, or green cards based on their needs and eligibility as survivors of domestic violence and other forms of abuse.

After I became a mom in 2016, I felt compelled to focus my career on supporting mothers and aspiring mothers—in the workplace, in society, and with their mental health. I advised and coached numerous new parents returning to work after parental leave, moms who were considering a career shift because they were afraid to ask for more flexibility at work, and other women struggling with the transition to motherhood. To become certified as a perinatal mental health practitioner, I sought additional training from the leading nonprofit Postpartum Support International, where I learned that up to one in five women experience a perinatal mood and anxiety disorder (PMAD) like prenatal anxiety or postpartum depression during pregnancy and through the first year of the child's birth. Of course, women can and do experience mental health struggles at any point in their lives, and if a PMAD is untreated, symptoms can last well beyond the perinatal phase.

Ultimately, I founded my private practice as a social worker (I'm licensed to provide clinical therapy in New York, New Jersey, Connecticut, and, via telehealth, Florida), through which I help women in their 20s through 40s, addressing stressors related to romantic relationships, family dynamics, careers, pregnancy, fertility, parenting, and more. I work with employee benefit programs to coach employees navigating the integration of work and motherhood. I frequently speak about issues like working parenthood, maternal mental health, and gender equity for corporate workshops, at various community events, and in the media. Supporting millennial moms and young women through life transitions is my passion, and I am privileged to be able to counsel and support women at vulnerable points in their lives as my job. I've witnessed the ways in which mental health can affect not just our moods but also our interpersonal relationships, our careers, our physical health, our identities, and more, and how important it is to have the right kind of coping mechanisms and resources to survive struggles.

I hope this context reflects how deeply I understand that mental health matters. And mental health during the menopause transition matters, in many ways.

We all know that anxiety, moodiness, and other mental health disorders affect quality of life in the present moment. Fortunately, for our generation, mental health has become a lot more destigmatized than in decades prior and most of us recognize the value of getting support during challenging times. Seeking help for these issues can improve both current quality of life and risk of other conditions down the road. And of course, our mental health plays a foundational role in a big transition like menopause. Mood issues during menopause can even impact (and increase the risk of) chronic and other health conditions.[121]

For now, let's discuss what mental health can look like in two phases: before the menopause transition and then during.

But before we do, I will put on my therapist hat and invite you to get comfortable. If you're able, you may want to place both feet on the ground. Consider putting one hand on your belly and one hand over your heart. Take a deep breath, inhaling through your nose and exhaling through your mouth. Focus on your breath and take it slow. Inhale. Exhale. Notice any thoughts that arise and try not to judge them. Just focus on your breathing. Take two more deep breaths just like that. Inhale. Exhale. Inhale. Exhale.

It's natural to feel overwhelmed by all this talk about menopause and the myriad struggles women may face while navigating it. My hope is that this book will help you feel less overwhelmed and less clueless. Because I'm right here with you. From the bottom of my heart, I hope you begin to feel more prepared and more empowered.

Ready? Let's explore together.

MENTAL HEALTH BEFORE THE MENOPAUSE TRANSITION

Many millennial women I know express fear and worry when just thinking about menopause. "I'm totally dreading that phase of life," a woman born in 1980 told me. "I am terrified! I don't want to be old and dried up," complained a friend born in 1987. "I am concerned about not having the right resources available when it happens," shared a woman born in 1984. "I associate menopause with medical risks that come with getting older, and I'm scared," reflected a woman born in 1985.

There's really no other way to say this—women's anxiety regarding aging is raging.

Anxiety can be thought of as a physiological response to an unknown risk. When we feel unprepared for something, we feel vulnerable. You may have experience with anxiety manifesting itself in the form of a pit in your stomach, a racing heart, irritability, teariness, and/or jitters. Anxiety can impact our sleep, our ability to concentrate, our libido, our overall happiness and well-being, and more. Anxiety can be mild and situational ("I'm anxious about this big project due next week") or debilitating and reflective of a disorder as characterized by the *Diagnostic and Statistical Manual of Mental Health Disorders* (DSM-5), including generalized anxiety disorder (GAD) or panic disorder. According to the FDA, anxiety disorders affect up to 40 million adults yearly, with current stats reflecting that women are more than two times as likely as men to develop an anxiety disorder in their lifetime.[122]

On the one hand, women these days may be more likely than in prior generations to access treatment for their mental health, which is a welcome shift but does skew diagnostic statistics. As proffered by a 2021 study, higher rates of anxiety disorders may be reflective of actual changes in symptom levels or just could be due to a "generational change in recognition of and willingness to report symptoms of mental illness."[123]

On the other, maybe being a millennial woman is simply really stressful. The 2023 State of Women Report from theSkimm, based on a study of 4,500 women conducted by The Harris Poll, showed that the majority of millennial women feel they are always adjusting their lives to accommodate others and they feel concern about the societal expectations around the unpaid labor/mental load that women are responsible for.[124] And perhaps it actually is harder to be a millennial mom than moms in prior generations, as posited in excellent 2024 essays by Hannah Seligson for *The New York Times* and Stephanie Hallett for *HuffPost*; in "Millennial Moms Don't Have It All, They Just Do It All," the latter author wrote: "We work more than previous generations of mothers, and we spend more time parenting our kids. We are at capacity all the time, even with the trappings of professional flexibility."[125] It's no wonder we're feeling anxious!

I see this all the time in my work and my personal life. The women I know are overwhelmed, to say the least. "You need to put your oxygen mask on first and carve out time for yourself," I often advise, and then go a full day without being alone even while peeing (Hey, do as I say, not as I do ... Therapists are people, too!) I used to bring my laptop to the dentist to catch up on emails in the brief moments my eyes weren't closed, telling the hygienist it was so relaxing just to sit back, no matter the dental drill scraping. I know women who have had emergency appendectomies and genuinely described their hospital stays as a welcome break from packing lunches and doing bedtime. One woman born in 1985* recently reflected of her breast biopsy experience: "It was so nice to be able to lie down in a quiet room and just focus on my breathing."

Our anxiety is not good for our health. And anxiety is not the only mental health issue with which women, especially millennial women,

---

* Dear reader, that woman was me!

are currently struggling. A study published in 2023 revealed that throughout the beginning of the COVID-19 pandemic, millennials (and Gen Zers) rated worse than older generations regarding not only generalized anxiety disorder but also major depression, perceived stress, loneliness, quality of life, fatigue, and other mental health indicators.[126] Also in 2023, researchers at the nonpartisan, nonprofit organization Population Reference Bureau found: "Millennial women's well-being in the United States has been negatively impacted by the changing social, political, and economic climate of recent years. While the data show the stark impact of the COVID-19 pandemic on young women's immediate well-being, our generational analyses show that many of these same patterns [for millennials] existed long ago."[127]

You may be reading all this and thinking: *Well… shit. I'm already anxious given everything I'm dealing with in my life and in this world, and now menopause is on its way, which will make me feel even more crappy and will further affect my mental health on top of everything, and I'm going to have to advocate for myself to get proper care but I don't know how to do that because it's scary, and I can't control when menopause will happen to me, and I can't control how menopause will affect me, and I can't control how hard it is to be a woman in general, and, and, and … Oh my god, I'm totally buggin'.*

I understand. Inhale. Exhale.

Now, consider what one of my own therapists once told me: Worry is the illusion of control. It's true we cannot control a lot here, like the fact that menopause is inevitable and may cause changes to our bodies and moods. But in reality, we don't need to control something to survive it or even thrive during it. We need support.

And fortunately, support is available.

If you're feeling like your worries (related to menopause or otherwise) are interfering with your daily life, or that your mood has been lower than usual lately, you may wish to seek professional help.* Peer and community support can also be invaluable during challenging times. Talk to friends or loved ones about how you're feeling. Sometimes saying a worry out loud (and labeling it as a thought or feeling, not as something that identifies you) can really help dismantle its impact. Ask for help. I know seeking help is not always easy, but you deserve it.

And don't discount the support you can provide to yourself. There are many great journals and workbooks available.** Talk to yourself the way you would a friend and treat yourself with kindness. Check out some self-compassion practices and exercises from Dr. Kristin Neff.***

Finally, remind yourself that when it comes to menopause, by reading this book, you *are* taking control to the extent that you can by preparing yourself. Menopause may still be the unknown, but you have support literally at your fingertips. By reading this book, you

---

* If you need immediate help, please call 911 in an emergency. There are also free 24/7 hotlines available in the United States like the National Maternal Mental Health Hotline (1-833-TLC-MAMA) and the Suicide and Crisis Lifeline (988). The provider listings available from Postpartum Support International (https://psidirectory.com/) or the Inclusive Provider Directory (https://www.inclusiveproviders.com/directory) or Pro-Choice Therapists (https://www.prochoicetherapists.org/) are some of my favorite resources.

** Some good ones include: *Reclaim Your Life: Acceptance and Commitment Therapy in 7 Weeks* and *Retrain Your Brain: Cognitive Behavioral Therapy in 7 Weeks: A Workbook for Managing Depression and Anxiety.*

*** Available at https://self-compassion.org/self-compassion-practices.

have been equipping yourself with information and options. You are strengthening your self-sufficiency by learning about resources. You are not alone.

MENTAL HEALTH DURING THE MENOPAUSE TRANSITION

Let's move on to how a woman's mental health may be affected as she enters the menopause transition. What can we expect? I get questions on this topic often from women who are anxious in anticipation:

- "Will it be like PMS × 10?"
- "Will I be an emotional mess?"
- "Will I even recognize myself?"

Again, I understand that a sense of control is comforting, but in truth, we can't know exactly what to expect when we're expecting menopause in regard to mental health or other symptoms. As you now know, every woman's experience with menopause is different. And the way we approach menopause mentally and emotionally can impact our experiences physically. "The mind and body are not separate," explained Dr. Kathy Casey, the acupuncture and Eastern medicine provider. "If you have a story in your head, your body will act that out. How we feel about this natural life transition will play a big role in how we navigate the shifts, and so when our perceptions—as well as societal perceptions—affect us, our biochemistry will respond."

Because we've been conditioned to fear aging and menopause, and because we're generally ignorant about it, women don't usually talk to themselves nicely about this change. From those in perimenopause, I frequently hear sadness regarding a shift in identity, a loss of youth:[128]

- "I don't feel old enough to be in this phase of life."
- "I liked being young and feeling free and now I feel like I'll never have that again."
- "I'm grieving the life I used to have" or "the kids I didn't get to have now that I'm losing my fertility."
- "I feel caught off guard, like I wasn't prepared. I feel out of control over my own mind and body."

And such narratives are not exactly mood boosters. Meanwhile, hormones like estrogen and progesterone affect our neurotransmitters like serotonin (which helps stabilize our moods) and dopamine (which helps with feelings of pleasure and satisfaction). And we know that during the menopause transition, our hormones fluctuate. Accordingly, women can experience heightened symptoms of premenstrual syndrome (PMS) or its more severe version, premenstrual dysphoric disorder (PMDD), like depression, irritability, and other symptoms of psychological distress.

Remember that menopause symptoms are not universal. Some menopausal women do not experience mental health (or other) symptoms at all. But certainly, many women do, particularly in the later phase of perimenopause while approaching the final menstrual period. And that can feel very difficult.[129] "My mind went to a really dark place," healthcare attorney Susan Frankel recounted of her menopause transition. "I started to feel different by about 47 or 48, but my menstrual cycle hadn't changed and menopause wasn't at all on my radar. But something definitely shifted for me internally, and only later I realized I was in perimenopause."

Frankel described crying "all the time" and being affected "by everything, way more than was warranted." She shared: "I felt crazy. I really felt like I was losing my fucking mind. I couldn't function." She also was simultaneously experiencing "crushing fatigue and brain fog" in addition to family issues that "caused a lot of stress."

Frankel's rough experience is not unique. Kara Cruz, the California licensed marriage and family therapist first mentioned in Chapter 3, often hears similar sentiments. Through her psychotherapy and wellness practice, Cruz provides clinical and psychoeducational services to perimenopausal women in both group and individual settings. These women tend to experience a range of anxiety and depression symptoms, including rage, shame, irritability, low energy, low motivation, feeling unworthy, and more. Cruz told me that her clients often express: "I wish I had been warned that perimenopause is like a second puberty, that I wasn't imagining all these changes or going crazy," and "I wish I had known earlier that perimenopause was even a thing!"

Perimenopause, we now know, is indeed a thing, and is in fact a vulnerable period of time when it comes to mental health. While depression is not a universal symptom of the menopause transition, menopause *is* a period of increased risk of depressive symptoms. According to The Menopause Society, perimenopause and the years just following menopause are periods at which women experience depression at twice the rate of that at other life stages like premenopause.[130] Other research shows that women are up to five times more likely to experience a major depressive episode while in the menopause transition and shortly after menopause.[131] Women at particular risk of high depressive symptoms include those who are Black, those with low educational levels or high body mass index, and who use alcohol and tobacco.[132]

Depressive symptoms include feeling sad, empty, or hopeless, experiencing a loss of interest in things and activities that used to bring joy ("anhedonia"), low energy, the inability to concentrate, feelings of worthlessness, or thoughts of suicide. There is more research available related to menopause and depression vs. anxiety, but as I like to tell my clients, anxiety and depression are like cousins: they are closely related and often together. Symptoms like hot flashes and poor sleep are also risk factors for depressed mood in perimenopause,[133] and, probably predictably, women who experience more severe menopause symptoms, including vasomotor symptoms, tend to also experience more severe symptoms of anxiety[134] (I think it's to be expected that a woman who has intense physical symptoms feels anxious about them).

"Perimenopause is actually the highest risk time for a mood disorder in the reproductive lifespan," explained psychiatrist Marra Ackerman. "This is not discussed nearly enough!" A few studies have highlighted the connection between perimenopause and major depression (and suicidal ideation and suicide),[135] but I agree—we need more attention to this issue in order to recognize it and help women enduring symptoms. And fortunately help can come in a variety of ways, including medication like SSRIs or SNRIs, behavioral modifications, and talk therapy, including cognitive behavioral therapy. "I often see improvement from using psychoeducation as an intervention; telling the patient that she is experiencing perimenopause, that it is temporary, and that she has options for treatment can be very worthwhile," Dr. Ackerman noted.

Why might a woman experience a mood disorder during the menopause transition? "Hormones clearly play a *huge* role in women's moods," per Dr. Ackerman. She pointed out that postmenopause, midlife females' depression rates tend to decrease to return to about the same level as that of midlife males.

A systematic review published in 2023* summed up the risk factors for developing depression or anxiety during the menopause transition as follows: vasomotor symptoms like hot flashes and night sweats, a history of major depressive disorder, neuroticism (a personality trait through which people experience negative emotions like anxiety, anger, or feeling threatened), stressful life events, and low financial or educational status can be major risk factors; minor risk factors include a lack of social support, being single or divorced, having a negative perception of aging or menopause, and a history of premenstrual syndrome/premenstrual dysmorphic disorder.[136]

---

* If you choose to read any of the scientific sources cited in this book, I'd recommend this one, "Does menopause elevate the risk for developing depression and anxiety? Results from a systematic review" from *Australasian Psychiatry*. The authors reviewed studies from throughout the world and their conclusions are clearly articulated. Admittedly, I did smile ironically upon reading in their introduction: "Perhaps surprisingly, no review of whether menopause elevates the risk of developing major depression and/or anxiety has previously been undertaken." Um, LOL. I am definitely not surprised. As we learned, too few researchers, policymakers, healthcare providers, and people in general seem to care about this issue. Anyway, these researchers did engage in the review, and for that we should all be grateful.

I am a therapist who primarily works with women experiencing anxiety and/or depression mood symptoms. I am also a woman who has personally experienced anxiety and depression. So, for me, the main takeaway from this review is to be aware to get prepared: If you have a past history of depression and anxiety, a history of postpartum depression, and/or an adverse perception of menopause (which, as discussed in Chapter 4, is basically what we've all been told to have by the media), you may be more likely to develop mood disorder symptoms during menopause.

Specifically, it has been found that a "prior depressive episode—particularly if related to reproductive events—is the strongest predictor of mood symptoms or depression during menopausal years."[137] Women with a history of depression are up to five times more likely to have a major depressive disorder diagnosis during menopause.[138] Relatedly, women with a previous history of both anxiety and depression have been found to "have the greatest risk for low quality-of-life during midlife."[139]

If you've never experienced a mood disorder, you seem to be at lower risk of experiencing one during the menopause transition. "It's relatively rare for someone with no history of depression or anxiety to suddenly develop a severe case of it at menopause," Dr. Hadine Joffe, a women's psychiatry expert, told Harvard Medical School's publication in 2020.[140] However, it should be noted that really, no one is immune. Mood symptoms can pop up for all women in the menopause transition. A 2021 research review revealed that "among women who present with depression during the transition, 16 percent were experiencing it for the first time;" according to the American Psychological Association, the reasons why "are varied, including hormonal shifts related to relevant brain pathways, life stresses, and insufficient sleep brought about by perimenopause and menopause symptoms."[141]

Let's unpack these symptoms and factors a bit further. About 4 in 10 perimenopausal women experience mood symptoms similar to premenstrual syndrome.[142] The phrase "Not feeling like myself" is commonly used by perimenopausal women, who associate the feeling with "anxiety, vigilance, fatigue, pain, brain fog, sexual symptoms, and volatile mood symptoms," according to a 2024 study.[143] A 2024 UK-based study found that perimenopause is a period of increased risk for other psychiatric disorders like bipolar disorder: Participants without previous history of mania were over two times as likely to develop mania for the first time during perimenopause than later reproductive stages (echoing an association between risk of first onset mania and the first few weeks postpartum after childbirth).[144]

If you feel cranky, distracted, teary, or simply unlike yourself, it may indeed be because your hormones are functioning differently than they used to. Perimenopause is often described as emotionally chaotic.[145] Some women with experience overcoming mental health struggles report feeling like they are no longer emotionally resilient when menopause symptoms begin or that they've lost their ability to deal with stressors (of which there are usually many).

Many women who have been through perimenopause have described it to me as a time when they felt wild waves of rage or extreme irritability, which would come in surges and which they could not control. "I would be in the best mood and then suddenly snap and feel like a wicked demon had taken over," recalled my family friend who was born in 1953 and experienced early menopause when her children ranged in ages of 1 to 10 years. "I hated yelling at my kids. The mood swings were the primary symptom for me, and they really took a toll."

The effects of changing hormones on how you feel physically can make you feel emotionally bad, too. You may feel embarrassed by having hot flashes during work or stressed about how your body, skin, or hair is changing. You may feel exhausted and like you want to withdraw socially, yet self-isolation is likely not going to be helpful to your mental health. And if you've ever experienced a trauma—whether sexual abuse, physical abuse, or emotional abuse (including workplace sexual harassment even without physical contact)—research shows that you may be particularly susceptible to physical symptoms like hot flashes and sleep disturbances.[146] Put simply, physical and mental health symptoms can continue to exacerbate each other.

While internally your hormones are all over the place, externally life is still happening. And life for women, we already know, can be stressful. As summarized in a 2023 article for the American College of Obstetricians and Gynecologists by Dr. Nazanin E. Silver, a psychiatrist and OB/GYN, perimenopause is a time "when life's pressures can be greatest. Many people in this age group are managing demanding jobs, raising younger children or sending older children off to college, and caring for aging parents. All of this stress can add to mental health challenges."[147]

Ugh. Can women ever catch a break?

I think so, actually, if they know what may be coming their way. It's not that women should try to try to avoid or control anything, which may be (and likely is) impossible. Rather, they can prepare themselves to navigate challenges with the right support systems in place and to recognize when they may need to seek out additional support.

HOW CAN MILLENNIALS PREPARE?

Consider Medication

As discussed in detail in Chapter 6, MHT can improve the physical symptoms of menopause (which may in turn alleviate mental health symptoms). And hormone therapy may specifically help with mood symptoms for perimenopause, too. There is evidence that estrogen can help regulate mood by impacting neurotransmitters and other physiological factors that are related to reward processing and motivation.[148] Specifically, transdermal estradiol therapies have been shown to significantly help with depression symptoms in perimenopausal women compared with placebo.[149] Anecdotally, several women have told me that they almost immediately felt less teary or irritable upon starting hormone therapy and had no need for other medications like SSRIs. But, more research needs to be done to clarify the efficacy and optimal timing of hormones on treating menopause-related mood symptoms. And, not everyone is a candidate for MHT or wants to pursue it.

Fortunately, there are other ways to improve mental health and other menopause symptoms.

We've talked about how certain SSRIs can be prescribed to alleviate hot flashes and can be used safely even by breast cancer patients. They are most commonly used, actually, to treat depression and other mood disorders like anxiety. So, they can be helpful for both the physical and mental health menopause symptoms, in addition to or as an alternative to hormone therapy. Some women report improvements in their mental health upon taking menopausal hormone therapy. But there's no shame in also needing an antidepressant like an SSRI or other interventions like psychotherapy to help with symptoms during this life stage.

"Personally, if I could do anything differently, I would have started menopausal hormone therapy and an SSRI much earlier," Frankel told me. "Some women feel much better emotionally once they begin hormone therapy, but some women, like me, need the additional help of an antianxiety/antidepressant for mental health." Frankel shares her journey so openly because she believes that doing so helps destigmatize these issues. I appreciate that, and I agree. In that spirit, I will share a bit of my own mental health journey.

By the time I was in my late 20s, I had tried a few different forms of therapy, including talk therapy and medication like SSRIs, to treat the anxiety and depression I had experienced for years. Knowing that a prior history of mood disorders is a risk factor for a perinatal mood and anxiety disorder (just as we now know it is a risk factor for depression or anxiety during perimenopause), I spoke with my OB/GYN about all of my options before trying to get pregnant.

I wanted to mitigate my risks and feel as good as possible. She referred me to a psychiatrist specializing in reproductive health, who helped me modify my treatment approach with a new-to-me type of SSRI that ultimately worked better for me, as well as a referral to a therapist who practiced cognitive behavioral therapy (CBT, the kind I primarily provide now).

I feel incredibly fortunate that my subsequent perinatal experience with each of my children was extremely positive. Despite my mental health history, I never suffered from a PMAD. I hope this gives you hope that, even if you have a history of anxiety or depression, you are not necessarily destined to have a difficult mental health journey while experiencing menopause.

Gather a Support Team

If you're a Marvel fangirl like I am, you will appreciate this: Avengers, assemble—it's time to build a team.

It would be impossible to parse out what exactly helped me during my perinatal time (the medication, the CBT, the open dialogue about my mental health with my healthcare providers, partner, family, and friends)—but I don't believe I have to. Instead, I believe it was the combination of the social supports I pursued and received that set me up for success. And social support/positive affirmations are also a known protective factor against developing menopausal depression and anxiety.[150]

So regularly see your OB/GYN as well as your loved ones and peers to discuss how you are feeling and get the help and support you need. "Once I started talking to my friends about how I was feeling, we realized we needed to keep sharing and supporting each other," reflected Frankel. "It has been so helpful to have each other's support."

The *Australasian Psychiatry* 2023 systematic review confirmed counseling/psychological therapy is a protective factor against developing menopausal depression and anxiety.[151] Cognitive behavioral therapy, in which one practices noticing her thoughts and cognitive distortions, reframes them to more neutral or positive interpretations, and modifies her behaviors to implement better coping strategies, can improve perimenopausal women's mental health and other symptoms.[152] CBT is increasingly recognized as a therapeutic tool available for the perimenopausal population at hospital centers like UCLA, which are offering much-needed holistic care for women in this phase of life.[153] It can be used as a complement to medication like hormone therapy or on its own, to help women manage the distress they may feel due to their symptoms.

Therapists can help assess how perimenopause symptoms may be impacting mood or impairment in functioning on a social or emotional level. You can stay in tune with your emotions by keeping track of them in notes on your phone or in a notebook if you're old-school and like to handwrite. Therapists can offer suggestions for apps, journals, or prompts to fit your preferences and make it feel less like homework, and then point out things you may not have known or seen. "The brain fog was extremely scary when it started happening to me. My therapist was the one who told me it's a common perimenopause symptom," a friend born in 1981 told me.

Since becoming better educated in menopause, I have noticed a pattern among a few of my clients' reported mood symptoms. When I inquire about changes to their cycle and/or suggest they see a menopause specialist, they have received confirmation they are in perimenopause, which hadn't occurred to them or ever been mentioned before. Through my studies, I learned about a screening tool for perimenopausal depression called the Meno-D, which is helpful for tailoring treatments to women in perimenopause.[154] I now teach other clinicians about resources like these in addition to using them with clients to better assess what is going on with them and what they may need to feel better. I am so glad I can now be a part of women's menopause care team.

In addition to psychoeducation and support, there are various therapeutic techniques that mental health practitioners can use to help women experiencing the menopause transition. For example, in her practice, Cruz uses CBT as well as somatic approaches, behavioral activation techniques, and EMDR (Eye Movement Desensitization and Reprocessing, a psychotherapy technique to help people heal from trauma) to alleviate her clients' menopausal mental health symptoms. She emphasizes that support groups and group activities involving movement like dance or sports can enhance feelings of social connectedness, safety, and community.

"Ultimately," she acknowledged, "menopause is a medical issue. So, a lot of the work I do with women involves empowering them to get the medical care they need and deserve, including by referring to a specialist or support group or helping them feel confident when seeking care."

Advocate for Yourself

I, too, focus a lot of my counseling practice on helping women assert themselves, in connection with healthcare and beyond. Far too many women struggle with asking for what they need out of fear of being a bother because women in our culture are conditioned to acquiesce and be easygoing. This is not only unfair but also potentially dangerous. Women who prioritize others' needs before their own are not getting their needs met. Recent research has confirmed that empowering self-management strategies can be extremely helpful for women in the menopause transition, given all of the biopsychosocial factors at play during midlife.[155]

"Women at midlife have been told for too long: 'Oh, it's natural to be stressed. Have some wine and a vacation,'" Dr. Brittany Barreto, the FemTech expert, described. "They've been unheard and gaslit, and the healthcare approach has got to change." Agreed Mama Beasts' Antoinette Hemphill: "It's women's way to be accommodating, to write off not feeling their best as 'just life.'" But, she urged, "we must break through that wall and recognize that we are worth the effort to feel our best. And it *is* going to take effort to figure out your particular perimenopause puzzle, to find what works best for you."

It may be especially hard for women of color to assert themselves because of potentially racist or patronizing responses. Veronica Eyo, LCSW, EdD, a California-based therapist and fellow Fair Play method facilitator and trainer who works with many millennial women of color, reports that several of her clients in the age range of 38 to 42 have noticed physical and emotional changes about which they asked their doctors. However, their OB/GYNs or primary care physicians typically tell them that the symptoms are due to being postpartum at their age. "But they'd been 'postpartum' for over one year. Their symptoms were just dismissed," Dr. Eyo described. "They had to continue to follow up or change doctors to finally be offered appropriate medication or hormone therapy."

We already know that women can be simultaneously postpartum and perimenopausal, and that Black women tend to suffer from menopause symptoms like hot flashes most severely—how frustrating that their doctors didn't! How lonely (and infuriating) it must have been for these women to ask for help and then get shut down. Fortunately, per Dr. Eyo: "Despite being dismissed by the healthcare system, they ultimately found support in family or other Black women who knew what the symptoms were. Through them, they felt validated and got suggestions for managing it." As their therapist, Dr. Eyo has supported them in reflecting on what perimenopause means for them—for this stage of life and for their future.

To all women, Hemphill cautioned: "If you seek treatment for menopause symptoms, you likely should be prepared to be a strong advocate for yourself." She recently went for a second opinion at a renowned women's health center that claims to specialize in menopause and was "dissuaded from hormone therapy, casually shamed about weight gain, and basically given a ridiculously oversimplified rationale" about what she was feeling. Hemphill believes that this experience is due to gaps in education and care practices that still persist in the medical community. Had she not been aware of this topic or self-assured, she said she would have walked out of that appointment completely defeated and full of self-blame. Instead, she walked out and made an appointment at a different practice, because she knows she deserves better care.

You do, too. It's time to channel your inner Elle Woods and advocate for what you need, for what you deserve. And you don't have to do it alone. A therapist like Cruz or Eyo or me can help. A community like Mama Beasts can help. We are in this with you.

Think About How You Think About Mental Health

I have a couple other thoughts on mental health I'd like to share. I want to emphasize that you do not need a diagnosis or to meet all the criteria of a diagnosis to get psychological support from a therapist. If you feel like shit, you deserve support. If you want objective reflections on stressful situations in your life, you deserve support. If you are going through a life transition—whether it's a new job, a new relationship, a new baby, a decision to be child free, a new chapter in your reproductive health, or anything else—you deserve support.

Menopause experts increasingly agree that optimal support during menopause combines psychological interventions aimed at depression with conventional therapies like medication.[156] If you need help accessing the mental health support you want or require during this transitional period, please reach out and I'll do my best to point you in the right direction and help you.

I also want to reflect on the word "crazy." We so often hear it about women. Women are often dubbed "crazy" when they're premenstrual, when they're pregnant, when they're postpartum, and now, we know, when they're in the menopause transition. Women are called "crazy" (or "aggressive" or "nags") when they dare ask for things they deserve like paid parental leave from their jobs or an equitable division of domestic labor within their homes.

Women who are "crazy" need therapy, per our cultural rhetoric, and that is partly why mental health treatment itself has been stigmatized for so long. I remember learning about "hysteria" as the first mental disorder attributable to women[157] (and yes, the term was derived from *hystera*, the root word for uterus in Greek, as is "hysterectomy"). From ancient times through the 19th century, women who experienced emotions including what we now think of as anxiety or sexual desire were called "hysterical" and subjected to horrible, misogynist "treatments" like forced sex. "Hysteria" was actually characterized as a psychological disorder in the older versions of the American Psychiatric Association's DSM until 1980—just about when the eldest millennials were born.

What if we stopped calling women "crazy" and started actually paying attention to how, when, and why they need help? What if we stopped shaming women for their sexuality or assertiveness? What if we stopped putting pressure on women to be perfect mothers (whatever the hell that means), to be agreeable all the time, to quietly endure pain while having sex, getting birth control, giving birth, or going through menopause? I have a feeling that would all be really helpful for women's mental health.

Just an idea though, no worries if not!

(Kidding. Obviously. Please, catch yourself if you use gendered, qualifying language like that. Your needs and ideas are *not* burdens!)

Other protective factors against developing menopausal depression and anxiety that have been recognized include healthy lifestyle and meditation/mindfulness. We'll take a comprehensive look at lifestyle, including sleep and exercise, in the next chapter, and more on meditation/mindfulness will come a bit later. (Hint: You got an introduction earlier when we went through the breathing exercise!)

Before we go on, consider taking a brief pause. Step outside, get fresh air. Or take a shower and sing at the top of your lungs to old Britney songs (just me?). Or call a friend who makes you laugh. Sometimes we need a little mental health break to recharge. Please, take what you need.

Chapter 9

BEAUTY, BODY, BRAINS—AND PERIMENOPAUSE

I looked at myself in the mirror in April 2020—a fairly uncommon practice while in quarantine and isolated from everyone except for my husband and two small and very needy children—and realized my hair had gone gray.

Not all over, but noticeably so. Certainly grayer than it ever had been before, and seemingly overnight. Was this stress-induced? Had I not noticed it before because I was busy with the busy-ness of pre-lockdown life? Was it just because I was getting older? What else was changing or about to change?

My hair was always one of my favorite physical features, I'll admit (ladies, give yourselves compliments—you deserve them). I have always worn it long and intend to indefinitely, even though more mature women often go for chic, shorter cuts. I wasn't prepared for it to change. Yet by the time I was 35 that month, I had enough grays to prefer it get dyed all over, regularly. (Much respect to my silver fox ladies, but I personally wanted to get back to my usual brown.) But it turned out to be hard to get the color quite right, to get it to look like it used to. It's possible if not probable that it never will go back to looking like it did when I was younger. And even though that's a bit sad, maybe that's OK. Because I, too, am not the same as I was when I was younger.

One of my favorite millennial comedians, Hannah Berner, has a bit about getting older she shares in her 2024 Netflix special, *We Ride at Dawn*: "Commercials are like, 'Do you have a fine line? *Ew*. Do you have a gray hair? *Disgusting*.'" She's talking about society's response to women turning 30. We all know how much harder it becomes as women approach 40, 50, 60, and beyond. We're told that our skin needs saving from sagging and that we need "mommy makeovers" to "get our bodies back." Again (and again and again), we're taught to resist and fear aging. "My mother never mentioned a word about menopause," a woman born in 1985 recently told me. "But she came over the other day with a shopping bag full of antiaging moisturizers and insisted I now needed them. It made me feel weird about getting older and wasn't the guidance I actually needed."

I'll give it to you straight. No matter how optimistic and affirming I want to be, I acknowledge that there are many things about aging and perimenopause that are, well, not great.

Let's take it from the top, starting with how your hair may change during the menopause transition. It's possible that my graying hair reflected a decrease in estrogen levels, though going gray is usually more due to genetics or, possibly, one's environment (and, probably, stress, which I was certainly experiencing at that time). Shifting hormones during perimenopause more commonly result in thinning hair on your head, which you may notice via a widening part or a receding hairline. According to Dr. Margo Lederhandler, a dermatologist based in New York, where the majority of her patients range in 30 to 50 years of age, hair often gets weaker.

It's also possible for perimenopause to bring you new, usually not wanted, facial hair. This can happen even after years of waxing, laser hair removal, and more. Fun! (NOT.) Typically, the new hair shows up in places like under the chin and above the lip. "I've also heard women complain about hair growth on new places like their cheeks," shared Dr. Lederhandler. "My laser technician was the one who first suggested my facial hair growth was due to hormonal changes," a woman born in 1983 told me.

That's not all that may be going on with your face. Remember how some people consider menopause to be like a second puberty? Well just like a first puberty, you may experience pimples during perimenopause. Per Dr. Lederhandler: "I often see hormonal acne, increased body odor, hyperhidrosis (increased sweating), dry skin, itchy skin, changes in skin quality or texture related to pore size or skin laxity, rosacea or facial redness, and/or more wrinkles due to decline in collagen and elastin." Upon noticing a facial patch of pigmentation I hadn't seen since being pregnant several years prior, I recently found myself googling: "Why do I suddenly have melasma?" and guess what the answer was? Hormonal fluctuations, i.e., perimenopause!

Added Dr. Leah Ansell, an instructor of dermatology at Columbia University and a medical and cosmetic dermatologist who practices in Rye, New York: "Probably the most common complaint I hear from women in the menopause transition is related to their lower face 'sagginess' or 'jowling.' I also see loss of skin luminosity or dull skin, etched lines and wrinkles, crepiness, volume loss, discoloration (accumulation of brown spots), worsening hooding of eyelids, loss of previously voluminous lips (due to bone resorption that occurs in the mouth and the soft tissue changes that occur in response), and other symptoms." She became interested in menopause-related care upon seeing patient after patient discuss the "exact same things and express shock and dismay at their changing appearance. They feel surprised and helpless. I help them tie together the symptoms by explaining the profound effects hormonal changes can have on our appearance and skin."

Let's continue with the rest of your body during perimenopause. After hot flashes, weight gain was the most-cited symptom that the 120 women I surveyed associated with menopause. "I've heard menopause leads to stubborn weight gain," a friend born in 1984 told me. "I've been in the perimenopause phase for years," a woman born in 1981 shared. "When will the belly fat stop?!"

Remember the hilariously real dressing room scene in 2002's *The Sweetest Thing*, where the characters played by Cameron Diaz and Christina Applegate jokingly long for their perky 22-year-old breasts and tight arms, compared with the droopier and looser 28-year-old versions? Well, consider your perimenopausal body more like the 28-year-old version—only now you're probably thinking, *Wow, if only I had realized how good it was at 28!*

I want to be clear that weight gain itself is not something I believe we should always fear or automatically assume is a bad thing. I certainly believe that women's value extends well beyond their appearance or body type, and that bodies in all shapes and sizes should be celebrated.

Still, I know it can be difficult to experience changes to your body that you didn't seek out or even know were potentially coming. I understand it can be tough to think, *My body is my own again!* after having babies, only to feel like everything you used to do to feel and look good in your own skin is no longer leading to the same results. Anita Mirchandani, a registered dietitian nutritionist and certified fitness professional, sees this trend often in her telehealth practice: "Women in their 30s and 40s often come to me and say, 'I feel weird. My body isn't doing what I've known it to do for many years. I can't lose the weight I've gained, especially in my midsection. It's making me feel stressed and crappy.'"

I've heard this a lot, too. Women often report to me that they don't recognize themselves in their midlife bodies. They describe no longer being able to fit into their clothes or that it feels like they've suddenly developed a pooch at their mid-section even after working hard on their core and abs post-giving birth. And they're not imagining it. The reality is, women usually do gain weight during perimenopause and after menopause.

Dr. Caroline Messer, the endocrinologist, confirmed that during the menopause transition, women typically gain up to 1 to 1.5 pounds per year. She explained that as estrogen levels drop, the body often becomes less responsive to insulin, the hormones that lowers blood sugars. To overcome systematic resistance, excess insulin is produced. Higher levels of insulin often translate to weight gain.

Dr. Messer added, "Insulin resistance is closely associated with a phenomenon called incretin resistance. Incretins are hormones produced by the gut which regulate hunger and satiety. Resistance to these hormones, including GLP-1 and GIP (the active hormones in medications like semaglutide and tirzepatide), can contribute to weight gain during the menopausal years by altering women's 'set points' for weight and modifying hunger and satiety signals."

Meanwhile, the rise of the pituitary hormone FSH during menopause may also be involved in weight gain. Plus, women tend to lose lean muscle during perimenopause, which slows metabolism and in turn can lead to weight gain. So, let's lean in to building up lean muscle!

We should also be beware of meno-belly—not just because we want to feel good about how we look on the outside, but also because fat at our tummy area can impact our health on the inside. Dr. Messer warned, "Fat deposition in the midsection is known as visceral fat and can raise the risk for a host of medical conditions including heart disease, asthma, breast cancer, and dementia."

I know this isn't wonderful news. But there *are* ways to prevent and mitigate weight gain. "As hormones fluctuate and the natural aging cycle of the body is at work, you may have lots of thoughts around lifestyle changes and drastic modifications," observed Tracy Lockwood Beckerman, MS, RD, a millennial registered dietitian and frequent expert contributor to media. She is also the author of *The Better Period Food Solution*, a guide to alleviating painful period symptoms through nutrition and improving health through every stage of the menstrual cycle. "But try not to take on an entirely different eating pattern that just doesn't suit you long-term or is too difficult to follow. This is a time to hone in on the things that we know are changing (like loss of both muscle mass and bones) and then better understand, assess, and enhance our intake of foods that will help us feel good."

There are also ways to work on being a little nicer to ourselves. If sweatpants are all that fit you right now, maybe you need to eat a little differently to ensure that you're getting appropriate nutrients and actually feeling full. Or maybe you need to go shopping for new clothes, since it's OK that your body changes over time (whose doesn't?!). The power of a mindset shift around body image is invaluable.

In connection with mindset... Let's talk about the brain. The good news is, beauty is on the inside, too; I hope you know that your self-worth should not be measured by the scale. Your intelligence and thoughtfulness are incredibly valuable and beautiful. The bad news is, your memory and brain function can be negatively impacted during the menopause transition as well. (You know the "This is your brain on drugs" commercials of the '80s and '90s? Well, your brain during perimenopause may similarly feel like a pile of mush on fire. Sorry!)

"Many women in their 40s come to me with similar complaints," noted Beth Silverstein, DO, neurologist and an assistant clinical professor at NYU. Common concerns include:

- "What's wrong with me?"
- "I can't recall things as quickly as I used to."
- "I feel confused, fuzzy, and foggy."
- "I have intense, throbbing headaches."
- "I can't retrieve words or names!"
- "I'm constantly blanking!"
- "Do I have dementia?"

To rule out any neurological causes like Parkinson's disease, other conditions like ADHD or untreated depression or anxiety, or underlying causes like poor sleep or nutrition, Dr. Silverstein will engage in detailed questioning, gather an extensive family history, and order blood work tests and cognitive computer-based testing as needed. Often, she finds that the underlying reason for these bummer brain behaviors is perimenopause.

A woman's drop in estrogen and other changes in hormones that occur during perimenopause can affect her brain both directly and indirectly,[158] including by driving inflammatory responses that can ultimately lead to neurological decline.[159] Women experiencing the menopause transition are more likely to experience forgetfulness and report feelings of brain fog than are premenopausal women.[160] The perimenopause-related effects on the body, including disturbed sleep or anxiety or other mood symptoms, can also impact memory and cognitive performance. For those of us women who have experienced "mom brain,"[161] in which we were already struggling to retrieve words or remember why we walked into a room (in part due to our total exhaustion), the perimenopause cognitive changes can feel like yet another heavy weight on our mental load.

"There is so much at play for a woman in this phase of life," acknowledged Dr. Silverstein. "I look at the whole patient. If her symptoms are due to perimenopause and there is nothing else going on, I refer to a menopause specialist who can help." The main takeaway, she wants women to know, is don't be afraid to seek help if you're struggling!

HOW CAN MILLENNIALS PREPARE?

Anticipate Physical and Mental Shifts

Preparation starts with knowing that some physical and mental shifts may occur sooner than you might have expected. "I always assumed menopause would happen in my 50s," shared Hemphill. "In some ways, I was correct in that the average age of menopause is 51, but I never understood that my symptoms leading up to actual menopause could start in my late 30s and early 40s. Since I wasn't focused on this, I wrote off a lot of symptoms as due to being stressed or not exercising enough." So many women I know do this, too.

But now we know better. Try not to convince yourself that your symptoms can't possibly be due to perimenopause. "I never knew how varied the symptoms could be," Hemphill admitted. "Night sweats were somewhat expected, but the brain fog, joint pain, and even dry hair—like, what?!" And you should know that treatment options are available for all of these.

In addition to seeking help for any bothersome or new symptoms, you can implement lifestyle changes—starting now—that will benefit your beauty, your body, your brain, and your overall health and well-being. Here are some suggestions.

Exercise

A wise woman taught us back in 2001 that exercise gives you endorphins and endorphins make you happy. And now we will learn that exercise can help with various health issues potentially impacted by menopause. "Get moving," Dr. Silverstein, the brain doctor, encouraged. "A sedentary lifestyle in which you are more stationary than not is not good for your brain or other areas of health." The more active you are during your midlife, the more you lower your risk of developing dementia later on.[162]

But keep in mind that being active doesn't necessarily mean going hard at the gym. "Move your body daily and focus on strength—not a number on the scale," advised Natalie Givargidze, the nurse practitioner and menopause specialist. "Building and maintaining muscle is crucial for women in their 30s and early 40s to help protect their bones through the menopause transition. Plus, the more muscle you have, the more fat you will burn as well."

Mirchandani explained: "There is no reason to overdo it. In fact, I see a lot of women who wake up early, work out, drink too much caffeine, don't eat enough all day, and then eat a big dinner, after which they are sedentary—this leads to weight gain." Instead, she recommends a combination of total body or core-focused strength training (including squats, chest presses, or box jumps) and walking for women in perimenopause, ideally about 20 to 40 minutes, five days a week. "I like to suggest swimming, yoga, and Pilates. Low-intensity steady state workouts are more effective than high intensity workouts in balancing cortisol and mood and burning fat. Also, any form of power walking is amazing!" Dr. Silverstein agreed: "Walking helps bring blood flow to the brain, which is great. I encourage brisk walks and water aerobics. It's never the wrong time to just start!"

Pilates and lifting weights can be especially helpful with building bone density, which is particularly important during late perimenopause and through early postmenopause.[163] Per the Bone Health & Osteoporosis Foundation, about 80 percent of the 10 million Americans with osteoporosis are women. Women become at higher risk as they approach menopause due to decreasing estrogen levels, which can cause lower bone mineral density and a decrease in bone mass. But the effects of lower estrogen on bones are somewhat preventable. The greater your bone density is when you reach menopause, the lower your chance of developing osteoporosis postmenopause, per the Foundation.[164]

"Bone is like living tissue. It sheds, it rebuilds," explained Lisa Schoenholt, the founder of Brooklyn Embodied, a virtual Pilates studio with in-person classes also available in the Westchester, New York, area. "When you add on weight while exercising, you are strengthening the bone. This is valuable even before menopause." In fact, all of the medical experts I spoke with for this book underscored the value of strength training at midlife.[165]

Ashley Austin, MD, a primary sports medicine doctor at the Hospital for Special Surgery in New York and a former Division I basketball athlete, confirmed: "Your bones will never again be as strong as they are in your 20s or 30s. That's a time when you feel invincible. But we won't feel that way forever. So start the strong foundation for bone health now. Now is the best time to get into a routine." The majority (more than 70 percent) of women in the menopause transition will experience musculoskeletal symptoms like joint pain, inflammation, osteoporosis, and cartilage damage, and a quarter of them will be disabled by them.[166]

To help prevent such symptoms, Dr. Austin emphasizes the importance of consistency (as even just 10 minutes a day, five to six days a week of strength training areas like the upper body can help with preventing injuries to the rotator cuff) and strengthening the hips/core, which can decrease injuries to the hip, knees, and spine. Variety is also key, since your body gets beat up with just one type of exercise. Dr. Austin suggests women focus on alternating high- and low-impact exercises, including HIIT workouts, sports, running, jumping, biking, swimming, barre, yoga, and Pilates. Additionally, she told me, working with exercise bands can improve bone density without high-intensity exercise or a full set of gym equipment or machines.

Exercising also includes working on your pelvic floor to build strong muscle mass before it starts declining during the menopause transition. "It's important for women in perimenopause to build a reserve of pelvic floor muscle strength," said pelvic floor therapist Dr. Sara Reardon. "You don't need to have a problem to implement a routine. And if you do have a problem, the earlier you get treatment, the better your outcomes will be. Learn how to engage your abdominal wall, breathe properly, and activate your pelvic floor. Be proactive!"

We are so often reactive in our approach to health, like having a date on the calendar that prompts us to implement an exercise routine or adopting certain workouts to resolve the impact of an injury. But this isn't the ideal way to prepare for the menopause transition. As Dr. Austin said, "Don't wait to train for some race or event. The training for life starts now."

Nourish Your Body

Millennials have always been told that women's bodies should look a certain way, whether that's heroin chic skinny or Brazilian butt lift full-figured (but also, still skinny). We've been told by magazines and social media to implement eating regimens like Atkins, keto, or the Special K diet. It's no wonder we have struggled with body image. But actually, what should we be eating to be healthy and strong, especially during the menopause transition?

I really appreciate Mirchandani's answer and general approach to eating, as instead of punitive it is intentional and well-balanced: "Food is fuel. Restricting calories is not the answer." Not only can consuming fewer calories cause the body to hang on to fat, but it is also, generally, unsustainable. "You have to find what feels good for you and your body, including what brings you joy."

Sarah Shealy, the nurse midwife and menopause specialist, also sees many women in midlife who restrict nutrition because they think it may help with losing weight. In actuality, they must eat more of certain kinds of foods to avoid deficiencies. "Many women are depleted of vitamins like Vitamin D and iron in the postpartum period and do not fully recover by the time they reach perimenopause, which further exacerbates inflammation and other symptoms." It's good practice to ask your primary care physician to do blood work panels at your annual visits to ensure that you are at a reasonable range for important nutrients rather than deficient.

Modifications to your diet can help, whether you *are* experiencing a deficiency or just to optimize your health. When it comes to the menopause transition and food, consider the following general guidelines.

Try to Add:
- Minimally processed, fresh food. Try to stick with fruits, veggies, and lean protein. Protein, per Dr. Austin, "helps keeps our muscles strong and helps prevent them from turning into fat." According to Lockwood Beckerman, "By maintaining muscle mass with protein, we can ensure we are supplying our body with adequate amino acids to protect our muscles and prevent them from declining."
  - » Animal protein is available in foods like grilled chicken or other poultry, fish, flank steak, or eggs.
  - » Plant protein is available in foods like legumes, edamame, and seeds. A plant-based diet like the Mediterranean diet can help lower cholesterol, which lowers cardiovascular disease risk.[167]

- Healthy fats, which can be found in foods like avocado, olive oil, and eggs.
  - » Mirchandani clarified that eggs contain what are considered heart-healthy fats, suggesting that "eggs can be eaten every day and at least two to three per serving."
- B12, which can be found in fish, poultry, eggs, lentils, nuts, seeds, or soy.
  - » Dr. Silverstein noted, "A vitamin B12 deficiency can be the reason behind memory loss or other issues. So make sure you're getting the right kind of B12-full-food to help with brain health."
- Vitamin D, which can be found in salmon, egg yolk, dark leafy greens, milk, mushrooms, fortified soy milk, or fortified cereal.
- Calcium, which can be found in whole food sources like dairy, almonds, and berries.
  - » Lockwood Beckerman explained, "Calcium-rich foods often also contain a smattering of other helpful nutrients like zinc, which helps your immune system, and polyphenols, which can reduce risk of chronic disease. They will help keep your body strong and balanced."
- Iron, which can be found in red meat, beans, oats, or white rice.
  - » Because periods can be so heavy during perimenopause, sometimes women end up being iron-deficient. Low iron can lead to restless leg syndrome and hair loss.
- Magnesium, which can be found in pumpkin seeds, peas, or quinoa.

- » Mirchandani told me that magnesium can help with digestion, stress, and blood pressure regulation.
- Omega-3, which can be found in various types of fatty fish, walnuts, spinach, or Brussels sprouts.
  - » Lockwood Beckerman added that these foods can "help us fight against health woes and can protect against depression, too."
- Water, which, per Dr. Silverstein, "helps with brain function. If you are dehydrated, you may have trouble concentrating or thinking clearly. So don't forget to hydrate!" (Cue me putting down my Trenta-sized iced coffee and grabbing a glass of water. Please get some yourself!)

Try to Avoid:

- Certain foods that tend to exacerbate your symptoms.
  - » For example, some women report that spicy foods can trigger hot flashes for them. Refined sugar can worsen symptoms like mood swings. I've also heard women experience new gastro reactions like diarrhea in response to the same foods they've always eaten. Try to keep track of what you've eaten before any spike in symptoms so that you can adjust as needed.
- Excess caffeine or alcohol, which "generally won't help with weight during perimenopause," Mirchandani warned. "But, you have to live your life."
  - » Unnecessary vitamins or supplements, as too much of anything can have detrimental side effects. Dr. Austin likes to recommend a daily multivitamin for women beginning in

their 20s. But, she cautioned against consuming supplements unless there is a known need: "There isn't a lot of good research or data on the efficacy of supplements."

Sleep Well

I absolutely love sleep. I think it's delicious. I want nothing more on holidays like Mother's Day than to catch up on rest and lounge in my bed. (I strongly recommend this as an alternative to hosting a brunch you have to organize and clean up for members of your extended family. You can tell them I told you to do this!) My family is one of night owls, so even though I tend to stay up late, I could regularly (and happily!) sleep past noon whenever I have the opportunity.

Sleep isn't just my personal favorite hobby, but also, it turns out, a protective factor against many of the potential perimenopause symptoms. So many of the experts I spoke with and studies I've read confirm that good sleep is pivotal to feeling good. Quality sleep is helpful for brain health, mental health, weight issues, skincare, and much more, including sexual function.[168]

"Impaired sleep can impact functioning on various levels," explained Dr. Nishi Bhopal, founder of California-based Pacific Integrative Psychiatry and of IntraBalance, a virtual training program for physicians and therapists on the importance of sleep. Poor sleep can impact not only quality of life and personal productivity but also public health and safety issues like driving and lead to more healthcare-related costs. In general, poor sleep can have really serious health risks. "Impaired sleep is associated with an increased risk of diabetes, stroke, coronary artery disease, and mood disorders," Dr. Bhopal pointed out. It also doesn't help with metabolism or burning fat, since inadequate sleep can lead to inflammation.

Furthermore, studies have found that restricted sleep (even just two nights of it) can significantly change the appearance of the skin and face for women aged 30 to 55.[169] I can personally attest to this, as during the week I wrote this very chapter, I got very little sleep due to a kid with strep who wanted to snuggle with mama and woke us up multiple times in the night. (Was it her fever-induced sweat or my perimenopausal nightly hot flash that had us both soaked? We may never know.) After two nights of this less-than-ideal sleep situation, I had multiple blemishes (ahem, zits). Instead of looking like a Noxzema girl, I looked a little green. It was no surprise to learn that chronic poor sleep quality is associated with increased signs of intrinsic aging, diminished skin barrier function, and lower satisfaction with appearance.[170] Beauty sleep is real, people!

Poor sleep can really mess you up mentally, too. As you may know based on experience, poor sleep can lead to a heavy feeling of fatigue, low energy, and—I can certainly confirm—a bad mood. You may be so sleepy during the day you need a nap to function—and if you have the time for that, please, tell me your secrets. Poor sleep can affect your memory, attention span, and ability to concentrate or make decisions. It can exacerbate mood symptoms like irritability or persistent crying, symptoms I see frequently in my perinatal clients. When I encourage (well, practically insist) that they get at least five consecutive hours of sleep while someone else tends to the newborn as needed, they feel immensely better, which is so rewarding to witness. For women in the menopause transition, poor sleep has been associated with depression and suicide.[171]

It's clear that sleep, like milk according to the ads of our youth, does a body good. You may have already been aware that good sleep is good for you, but now you know it's necessary. And while it may not be possible to completely avoid sleep-related issues with perimenopause, the severity of sleep disturbances (and in turn, many perimenopause-related symptoms) can be alleviated with certain behaviors. "Sleep impacts virtually every facet of life and health, including mental health, physical health, and social or interpersonal connections," emphasized Mollie Eastman, the founder of Sleep Is a Skill, a company that uses technology, accountability, and behavioral change to help people optimize their sleep. "Try to think of prioritizing sleep as investing in a (free) behavior that helps bolster and support all other areas, so that you can show up more powerfully everywhere else."

Both Bhopal and Eastman encourage implementing behavioral modifications to achieve healthy sleep. I always thought the key to sleep hygiene was going to bed at a consistent time, but they clarified that a consistent wake-up time is perhaps even more crucial (as it can help reset our rhythm for the day). Bright light in the morning, fresh air and time outdoors, and regular exercise are helpful daytime habits. At night, when it's time for bed, we can use blackout curtains, white noise machines, and/or cooling mattress toppers as needed to get into a good groove. In fact, it turns out that a cool (and dark and quiet) bedroom is ideal for sleep even if you don't experience night sweats.

Limiting social media and screen time before bed is really important to help you wind down before going to sleep. A phone's blue light can dysregulate our melatonin production, and what we're consuming on social can impact our mental health, even if we think we are doing it passively. To avoid the temptation of mindless scrolling, consider keeping your phone out of arm's length, maybe even in a different room (actual alarm clocks still exist, I swear!). If you do like some nighttime media as part of your routine, try reading from an e-reader with a warm color setting or listening to a meditative podcast.

Other pre-bedtime practices to avoid (that you likely already know but may need to be reminded of and held accountable to) include consuming caffeine and alcohol, which can disrupt sleep. The practice of stopping eating at least two hours before bed can be helpful for digestion, metabolism, and relaxing the body in time for bed. "I love granny dinner hour," Dr. Robbins has joked. And now I'm thinking the older women responsible for the early bird special trend were aware that an early dinner time slot helped them feel good as they went through menopause.

Back to sleep itself... The general recommendation of quality sleep is seven to nine hours for the average healthy adult. Which, honestly, *goals*, as the kids say. Meaning, probably more aspirational than attainable, at least for someone like me. I admit that I do not—yet—consistently get this amount of sleep. I myself am guilty of engaging in revenge bedtime procrastination, where, like many moms and women out there, I will stay up late doing "me time" things. In another life, I may have been a vampire. I knew I'd be close with Nicole Brujis, my stylist and best mom friend, when she described: "I come alive in the night." Like I said, I really (!) love sleep—but I also love my alone time at night. Everyone has the same 24 hours in a day as Beyoncé, and frankly, she's probably a tired and touched-out millennial mom like the rest of us, craving solo time where she's undisturbed and able to watch Bravo, organize her closet, eat some Häagen-Dazs, catch up with a friend through memes, or maybe even read.

So how can millennial women access the elusive magic of sleep?

"The first step is to make sleep a priority," encouraged Dr. Bhopal. "Many millennial women are so used to being tired or not sleeping well. When you're busy and overwhelmed, sleep is usually the first thing to go out the window." But seven to nine hours of quality sleep is clearly worth pursuing in midlife and probably always.

One way to approach it, as I counsel all my clients who have large goals, is to start small. The late, great Supreme Court Justice Ruth Bader Ginsburg once said: "Real change, enduring change, happens one step at a time." You don't have to flip a switch and immediately implement a lights-out curfew by 10 p.m. every night (though you could, and you go girl if you do), but you (we) could start with small steps. Start by being mindful about what's keeping you up late, challenging yourself to put something nonurgent off till tomorrow, and asking for support if you need the time for self-care.

Affirmed Dr. Bhopal: "Quality sleep is not about striving for perfection in a sleep routine, but rather about creating a lifestyle that works for your unique needs and supports your physical and mental health." And if you're struggling with doing so, or with any kind of regular sleep disturbance, do not wait to seek help. Maybe you need some emotional support for the mental load that is weighing on you. Maybe you need some tangible support at home, in the form of another caregiver putting the kids to bed or a partner loading the dishwasher (and actually running it and then putting the clean dishes away). Maybe you need logistical support at work in the form of a flexible schedule or commuting policy.

Maybe there is something physiological or health-related going on. Eastman pointed out that there are more than 100 sleep and wake disorders that can impact sleep. If you or your healthcare provider suspects a disorder like sleep apnea may be interfering with your quality of sleep (and in turn, adversely affecting your brain health and health in other areas), you can get a sleep study to confirm. "I often suggest sleep studies—whether at home or in a center—if needed," described Dr. Silverstein. "If sleep apnea is confirmed, depending on the patient, I suggest a mouthguard or provide a referral to a pulmonologist or ENT for further interventions."

Dr. Bhopal emphasized that getting your sleep evaluated early on by a professional can help prevent and reduce sleep-related issues from progressing. "Sleep issues are highly treatable!" she expressed. There are various treatment approaches, including behavioral (like cognitive therapy for insomnia, a structured program that is effective in about 80 percent of people, helping them identify and change the thoughts and behaviors that cause or worsen sleep problems while learning skills to reduce and prevent insomnia), medical treatments, and lifestyle modifications, all of which can help reduce sleep disturbances during the menopause transition. Poor sleep does not need to be part of your new normal. Help in various forms is available!

Get Prescriptions and Professional Healthcare as Needed

All of these lifestyle changes are useful as general guidelines, and of course you should speak with your own medical provider to get individualized advice for your particular needs. Be sure, too, to get appropriate care to rule out other health issues that may be impacting how you feel or look. For example, menopause is not connected to the thyroid, per Dr. Messer (who clarified that "thyroid levels do not change as a result of menopause"), but thyroid disorder symptoms can resemble some perimenopause symptoms, including changes to mood and/or weight, sensitivity to temperature that can seem like a hot flash, or changes in your menstrual cycle.[172] So providers like Dr. Silverstein frequently consider the thyroid when presented with such symptoms.

And of course, even if your symptoms are due to perimenopause and not some other medical issue, you deserve quality healthcare, including prescription medication if that helps you. For hormonal acne, for example, a dermatologist can prescribe topicals or oral medication if deemed appropriate. "I like to treat skin issues with a personalized, multimodality approach specifically tailored to a patient's skin and goals," explained Dr. Lederhandler. "That can include a combination of topicals, lasers, other devices that can stimulate collagen production (such as microneedling, microneedling with radiofrequency, or ultrasound technology), and judicious use of injectables (botulinum toxin, fillers, or biostimulators)." Skin treatments with retinol, available in over-the-counter forms or by prescription for higher concentration levels, can help improve skin appearance.

Topical estrogen creams for facial skin may also be helpful and are localized (so that they do not cause effects throughout the body and are generally deemed safe even for women with contraindications to systemic hormone therapy). Dr. Ansell said she hopes for more research on women at different ages using topical estrogen so that more data can become available about its efficacy and specific usages. As for systemic menopausal hormone therapy, Dr. Ansell often directly observes its profound impact on the skin. "I can almost always guess a patient is on MHT if she has certain skin quality that is somewhat unexpected for her age." Hormone therapy can also be helpful to alleviate a variety of beauty, body, and brain-related perimenopause symptoms, including brain fog, albeit indirectly.

There are other medications that can be useful at this time of life depending on your symptoms. For example, Dr. Messer explained, that beyond healthy eating and regular exercise: "The key to weight loss during menopause often involves incretin therapy to overcome systemic insulin and incretin resistance. Medications like semaglutide and tirzepatide help restore insulin sensitivity, allowing for weight loss and a simultaneous reduction in cardiovascular risk factors." I personally know a few postmenopausal women using semaglutide medications like Ozempic or Wegovy who report desired levels of weight loss and much-needed lower blood pressure, effects that have been confirmed in recent research.[173] Such medication can also be beneficial for one's mental health, as many women report feeling free from worrying about food. Keep in mind, though, as Mirchandani cautioned: "Drugs can be helpful but are usually temporary. It's ideal to figure out complementary practices that suit your lifestyle and routine so that you can maintain your health long-term."

Engage in Self-Care and Self-Compassion

Assuming long-term health is our goal, we have to take care of ourselves now. "If you prioritize yourself now, your health will be well cared-for later," Schoenholt of Brooklyn Embodied Pilates asserted. Many women I know in their 40s, 50s, and 60s agree that valuing one's own health and well-being is imperative. "Learn how to create time for yourself now, before it feels like life is swallowing you up," one midlife woman told me.

As a therapist who works with many high-achieving women, I consistently see that time for self-care is difficult to carve out. I get it; we are busy! But consider the costs of not investing in ourselves, of not learning how to manage our stress, or of letting ourselves get consumed by negativity or overwhelm. "We live in a hustle culture where women are constantly pushing themselves to do it all, for their kids, partners, parents, jobs," reflected Dr. Silverstein. "That may not necessarily cause dementia, but it surely leads to burnout, which is not good for physical or mental health." So please, take actual care of yourself!

Self-care includes seeking treatment for your health, and not just at your annual physical (though that's important, too, and should include regular screenings of your cholesterol to check in on cardiovascular disease risk, as discussed further in Chapter 14). It means taking the time to strengthen your pelvic floor to help with low back pain.[174] It means taking the time to engage in mental health therapy to learn effective coping mechanisms. It means taking the time to laugh with people who bring you joy.

And, I must add, it means figuring out how to be nice to yourself in regard to perimenopausal changes. I know it's not easy. We likely look different than we used to, and that can change be difficult, especially in the digital age. "Millennial women, as the generation who got social media in our teens and 20s, have so many photos of themselves out there on social media," reflected Kara Alaimo. "We have even more opportunities to scrutinize ourselves than women of past generations." Such scrutiny usually doesn't make us feel very good, and may be a huge factor in the rise of plastic surgery that took off along with social networks to achieve what she calls "toxic beauty standards" accessible only through heavy filters and expensive and sometimes risky cosmetic procedures.

I believe that feeling beautiful in whatever way works for you is important, and I also very much believe that inner beauty is even more important. We should build each other—and ourselves—up, not only for our appearances, but also for our inner qualities. Alaimo suggested sharing and liking unfiltered photos to start (at least, I'll add, remind yourself that what you're seeing is likely edited!). Another great idea is to comment about a woman's brilliance or that she's making a difference, instead of or in addition to a note complimenting her appearance. "These are ways we can start to help change negative norms, which will make spaces both online and offline healthier for women." I also like to encourage simply spending less time on the phone (though I know it's not actually simple. But it's worth trying!).

Midlife is a season of many changes that may not have been sought out, but it doesn't have to be miserable. Dr. Casey, the acupuncture and Eastern medicine provider, encourages women to consider menopause as a "second spring"; in Chinese medicine, she told me, the menopause journey is considered an awakening or even a new birth, a time "when women are able to use experience and knowledge to express themselves authentically and think of the aging process as an inward journey to wholeness." That mindset itself can be incredibly beautiful.

As my dear friend and partner in all things writing and witchcraft Drew Isserlis Kramer has expressed of aging: "My collagen is waning, but my chutzpah grows." I hope we can all move toward a feeling of acceptance. You may never again have the smooth skin, tight body, or sharp memory you had a decade ago, and that can be disappointing—but you *are* here, now. Too many women I know regret not appreciating the beauty, body, and brains of their youth. It's not too late to start.

Oh, and wear sunscreen.

Chapter 10

LET'S TALK ABOUT SEX

So far, I've talked about how perimenopause can bring with it physical changes like serious sweats, headaches, midsection flab, and fatigue, plus emotional and mental symptoms like the inability to concentrate, forgetfulness, and mood swings.

Do I make you horny, baby? Are you a sex machine?

If you're not exactly feeling DTF, I get it. In fact, I hear it all the time from my clients and friends. "My sex drive is already low," a woman born in 1984 told me. "I'm a mom of two kids, my job is intense, I'm always tired. I miss having regular sex and wanting to have more regular sex, but who has the time or energy?!"

I hear you, honey. The day-to-day grind of life at (and before) midlife can feel really tiring, which doesn't exactly make one feel sexual. And we all probably know what it's like to finally be in the mood, feeling yourself, and/or feeling your partner—and a kid walks in, demanding to know where the favorite stuffed animal is (tip: check deep down in between the sheets). Mood ruined!

Sex drive decreases gradually with age in both men and women. "As we age, our needs and desires and physical bodies change," explained Carli Blau, a sex and empowerment therapist and women's health expert licensed in New York and New Jersey. "Change is to be expected but does not need to be permanent. Good communication, self-exploration, and the support of a sex therapist can help."

Women are particularly likely to be affected by a decline in sex drive as they age.[175] Why? "There are so many variables that can affect libido for women in their 30s and 40s," reflected Dr. Alicia Robbins, the OB/GYN and menopause specialist. "Women at this phase of life tend to have needy kids, they're not getting enough sleep, they feel like their adult or alone time is limited." And then, when estrogen and testosterone start dropping during perimenopause, women tend to experience low libido as well as physical changes that make sex less pleasurable. "The biological changes can certainly lead to less interest in sex," per Dr. Robbins. "Women can experience less elasticity and less lubrication in their vaginas. The dryness and tightness are painful. And if you're having painful sex, then you're not having sex!"

If you're feeling vaginal discomfort, ensure that it's not due to other health issues like a pelvic floor dysfunction, urinary tract infection, or a yeast or bacterial infection. Your healthcare provider can help. You may want to use an at-home vaginal health test like those offered by Evvy, a biotech company with the mission to close the gender health gap by providing female healthcare services like vaginal microbiome tests.

Throughout my research for this book, I was reminded repeatedly by medical experts that the most powerful sexual organ is the brain. So if you're not in the mood, it could be related to your actual mood. Your low sex drive could be a side effect of mood disorder symptoms connected to depression—or to treatments for depression. Unfortunately, SSRIs (which, as discussed, can be incredibly helpful medications to alleviate symptoms of anxiety and depression as well as hot flashes) can make it difficult for women to get aroused or reach orgasm. You may also be feeling less sensual because you're less comfortable in your body; I hear every day, "I just don't look like I used to; my body image sucks and I don't feel sexy."

Let's not give up hope, girlfriends. Your libido may not be what it used to, but it can get back there—and be even better. Sex is an important part of physical and mental health, and can be really significant in relationships (including the one with yourself). Sexual activity, including masturbation, can even lead to stress reduction[176] and menopause symptom relief[177]—which may in turn lead to more sex! And of course, it's worth pursuing because of simple pleasure.

HOW CAN MILLENNIALS PREPARE?

Implement Some Sexy-Time Strategies

Let's set you up for successful sex. Your body is still a wonderland!

First, let's consider some things you can do to change your behaviors around sex, assuming you're not in pain but rather struggling with lower sex drive. Your body may be different, but you are beautiful and worthy of pleasure, in every single way. "It's imperative you get to know your body as it is now," encouraged Dr. Blau. Remember the advice we got as preteens to look at ourselves in front of a handheld mirror? Get the mirror back out! "And do speak to a healthcare provider about any changes—like growths or changes in smell—to rule out a medical condition."

Next, and you will probably not be surprised to hear this advice given what we covered in the last chapter: Get good sleep! It will help you feel better physically and emotionally. Poor sleep quality (not necessarily duration) has been associated with lower sexual activity and greater risk for female sexual dysfunction, especially for midlife women.[178] And literally spending more time in bed can't be bad for your sex life.

That said, don't be reluctant to get creative regarding when and where and how you have sex. My friends and I often laugh at the idea of sexy time after a romantic night involving lots of food (remember the *Sex and the City* episode where Charlotte runs to the bathroom with various tummy issues after an evening out?). You're likely tired and full, and that's OK! Consider having sex as soon as the babysitter arrives, in the shower, in the car, whatever works for you! Don't be afraid to lock the bathroom door (assuming the kids are safe elsewhere) and go for it. And remember that there are plenty of ways to get intimate with your partner that don't require penetration.

I work with many women in the postpartum phase who can't imagine reincorporating regular sex into their lives. But they usually report that once they do it, they want to do it more. So flex that muscle!

Communicate

Let's also strengthen your emotional connection through and regarding sex. Sex should not feel like a chore, but oftentimes women are thinking about chores and all the other things they have to do instead of spending time on sex. Studies have shown that women's disproportionate share of domestic or household labor (and related cognitive labor) is associated with women's depression, stress, burnout, overall mental health, and relationship functioning, including lower sexual desire. [179] In other words, when women perceive their partner as dependent on them, when they are overwhelmed by not just doing the domestic tasks but also thinking about them, when the division of labor is unfair… they are not in the mood for sex. (Duh!) "I want to want to have sex with my husband in theory, but in reality, I usually want to use any time I have to binge-watch *Suits* [or some other comfort show] in old pajamas while I get through the endless piles of laundry," more than one millennial woman has expressed to me.

Hope is not lost, though, because you can speak to your partner about what you need. "Raising the issue can feel intimidating for some people, but if you frame it as, 'I want to reconnect' or 'I want us to have better sex,' it can be really liberating," suggested Dr. Blau, whose therapy practice helps couples figure out ways to become reinvested in each other romantically. Meanwhile, through my work, I provide cognitive behavioral therapy, which has been proved to improve midlife women's sexual functioning. I often help women and their partners more effectively communicate about the mental load using tools like Eve Rodsky's Fair Play method,* so they can more equitably divide up the work and free up time for themselves, including for sex. It's truly worth talking about!

Consider Medical Care

And please—though I know it's not easy and can be embarrassing—speak with your healthcare provider about what's going on for you. After or in addition to some behavioral and cognitive adjustments, consider medication. "Many perimenopausal women benefit from testosterone hormone therapy," explained Dr. Robbins. It can help with libido and energy. However, she warns, "There is no FDA-approved testosterone formulation in the United States for women; it's available only in doses made for men." So yeah, we are back to Chapter 7 and wondering if anyone cares about us.

---

* *Fair Play* is a book, card game, documentary, and other media inspired by activist Eve Rodsky's experiences as the default (or "she-fault") parent and her well-researched findings, including that women are not biologically wired to be better at multitasking than men and that an organizational system of task ownership is more effective than avoiding actively communicating about domestic duties. Learn more at https://www.fairplaylife.com.

Dr. Robbins urged: "Ensure you are working with a qualified healthcare provider who can walk you through how to properly dose testosterone. Please do *not* get pellets from a med-spa or unqualified provider. It can have irreversible side effects if the wrong dose!" In fact, all of the certified menopause specialists I spoke with encourage women to avoid unregulated hormones in the form of pellets, which can be costly and quite dangerous and are not well-researched in women.

But under the right care, testosterone may be a game changer for your sex life (as can estrogen, which can help with the dryness and other physical factors). The International Society for the Study of Women's Sexual Health has guidelines for using testosterone therapy in perimenopausal women to treat hypoactive sexual desire disorder (HSDD), while calling for more research, especially on proper dosing.[180] Melissa Ferrara, a board-certified family nurse practitioner and the associate director of Maze Women's Sexual Health in New York, explained, "Topical testosterone is often a first-line option for women who have HSDD. We prescribe it in gel form that women usually apply on their leg (as one of the side effects can be increased hair growth at the site of application)." Ferrara reported that her patients often describe a boost in confidence upon taking testosterone, in addition to a higher libido. A September 2024 observational study also showed improvement in mood and cognition for women who use testosterone.[181]

Moreover, there are fairly new medical treatments available for women's low sex drive, which you likely have not heard of yet but about which we should all be screaming from the rooftops because they are not talked about enough. "Most women and most providers do not have any idea that there are two FDA-approved (nonhormonal) medications for libido," noted Dr. Robbins. An informal survey among my friends and own doctors confirmed that they are unaware. These drugs may not be appropriate for all women for a variety of reasons, but they are out there, and they are options for women. "It's not that they create spontaneous desire in women, but rather make you more receptive to sex, and help the body sort of fill in what was missing when it comes to libido," Ferrara explained.

One of the medications is an injectable called Vyleesi, a prescription medication for women who have not yet gone through menopause. It's not for women with uncontrolled blood pressure or known heart disease, and will not affect sexual performance, but it can help rekindle sexual desire and be used as needed. Ferrara described that Vyleesi works to help prime the body for sex and increases desire, in part by bringing blood to the genitals.

Another potentially helpful medication is called Addyi, which treats HSDD and is a pink prescription oral medication that must be taken once daily at bedtime to be effective. It is produced by Sprout Pharmaceuticals, a company founded by Cindy Eckert, founder of The Pink Ceiling, a firm investing in women-led healthcare businesses. Pink? Women-focused? Better sex? Sounds good to me!

Even if Addyi is not ultimately right for you, it nevertheless could be worth exploring as a potential option with your provider. In fact, you may be the one teaching your provider about it. "When it was first rolled out, it had a black box warning with alcohol. It was thought to put women at increased risk of feeling drunk and potentially fainting," Ferrara explained, alluding to one reason why many providers haven't been presenting it as an option to patients. "Now we know you can be taking Addyi and have 'normal' amounts of alcohol, and the warning has been removed. But the people who need to get the word out—like OB/GYNs and psychiatrists—are still not doing so as much as they should be."

It also doesn't help that—yet again—women are often not properly diagnosed with sexual dysfunction and in turn denied or never even offered treatment. I've heard stories where coverage of Addyi was denied by health insurance companies until the woman tried (and failed) marital counseling. *Excuse me?!* You know (and research shows) that if a man were to complain about sexual dysfunction or discomfort, he'd more likely and sooner get the help he needs.[182] One of my perimenopausal clients was astonished when her husband was quickly prescribed Viagra to effectively treat his midlife sexual struggles, while she has had to navigate various physical and emotional challenges impacting her sex life for several months. It feels wildly unfair, and it is (plus, testosterone prescriptions for women are not currently covered by most insurance plans in the US).

Dr. Robbins posited: "I think people in our society don't prioritize women's sex life or quality of life." In 2024, Eckert echoed as much to *People* magazine: "'When Viagra was approved for men's most common sexual dysfunction, it received rare fast track status and was FDA approved within six months. Addyi took six years. It tells you how little we value pleasure for women.'"[183]

Well, I value your pleasure. And I propose we continue these initially awkward but very necessary conversations with our providers, with our partners, and among ourselves.

Modify Your Mindset

Look, ladies, the reality is that we are not horny teenagers anymore. And that is OK. "There's nothing wrong with you if you don't want to have sex and nothing wrong with you if you do want to," Dr. Mandelberger, the menopause specialist, suggested. "Everyone is different. There is no medical need to have a libido and at this stage of life, it's natural to feel like so many other things are on your mind." *Um, yeah, like work stress, my kid needs me to fall asleep in his bed, plus I don't feel great in my bod*, you might be thinking.

Remember, though: If you do want to enhance your libido or change your sex life, treatment is worth exploring! Some treatment options can be behavioral modifications and a mindset shift. "I really want to dispel myths about sexuality and sexual functioning," said Ferrara. "You are not 'supposed to' want to have sex all the time, you do not need to have a feeling that you're always ready to go." Sometimes, she explained, sexual wellness and sexuality don't come (no pun intended) naturally. But that does not mean something is wrong with you. Ferrara put simply: "You shouldn't feel bad if you aren't multi-orgasmic the first time someone touches your clit."

You mean we shouldn't expect to always or easily feel the kind of euphoria hinted at in those '90s Herbal Essences commercials ("Yes! Yes! Yes!") or that Monica experienced while merely talking to Chandler about what she dubbed women's seven erogenous zones? That sure takes a lot of pressure off. According to Ferrara, only 30 percent of women orgasm from intercourse alone, a fact I am often teaching my clients (adults in their 20s, 30s, and 40s) who worry if they are "normal."

Still, pleasure should be accessible. And guess what? More pleasure may be around the corner, after menopause actually happens.

One benefit to menopause is, if you have a male sexual partner, you don't need to worry about getting pregnant. This usually comes as a huge relief to many women who have been consciously or subconsciously thinking about pregnancy for their entire adult life. As one woman very close to me who was born in 1930 unabashedly told me: "After I went through menopause, I felt very different—much lighter. It was wonderful. I didn't have to deal with my monthly cramps. And, it was such a load off to know I didn't have to think about birth control. I loved to fuck." (Yes, this quote is real, and it's spectacular.)

Another benefit is that as you age and hopefully become more in tune with your body upon reading books like these, you may feel more confident. I hope you do. You should be feeling yourself, literally and figuratively. Ferrara said one of her goals is to empower women to explore their own sexuality and sexual identity before linking that to a partner, and I love that for her, for all of us.

Your sexual confidence is still inside you. One might say it's like a genie in a bottle, baby. Come on and let her out.

Chapter 11

PERIMENOPAUSE AT WORK

By now we've learned that a lot of the issues we may or soon will be experiencing emotionally, mentally, and physically are potentially, if not probably, perimenopause at work.

So how does perimenopause affect us *at work*?

"I had my first-ever hot flash during a presentation I had been preparing to give for weeks," a friend born in 1977 told me. "It was intense." Given that hot flashes happen on average four to five times a day (with about a third of women having more than 10 per day and some women having as many as 20 per day),[184] this is a very real, potentially very difficult, thing you may have to navigate while working.

Several women I've spoken to have described suddenly dripping with sweat during a meeting. They find it embarrassing for a variety of reasons and struggle with inflexible in-office mandates during this phase of life. Many report wanting to leave their jobs or that they are contemplating early retirement because they're struggling with menopause symptoms at work. And with up to one in five women in the workforce currently in some stage of the menopause transition,[185] this is certainly an issue to which the workplace should pay attention.

While menopause is definitely not a disease, it does often involve symptoms that can make a woman feel ill or in need of care. Unfortunately, women tend to already struggle with requesting time off or accommodations for their health because they fear being considered a bother or risking discrimination. It's often hard enough for women to say "I need a sick day" and actually take it, and they may feel even less deserving or able to ask for one when it's needed due to menopause. As we know, menopause and other women's health issues do not get discussed enough and are still stigmatized in our culture.

Have you ever worked while sick with a cold? The flu? While pregnant and experiencing morning sickness or nerve pain? While freshly postpartum or breastfeeding? I would guess, given America's work-first culture and our shameful dearth of paid parental leave policies, yes. How was that for you? Probably not ideal for your health.

Potentially not ideal for your career, either. Sex and age discrimination are generally illegal in the United States due to federal law as well as local policies, but still very much occur in all sorts of industries. "We see discrimination in various forms," conceded Brittany Weiner, a millennial attorney and a partner at Imbesi Law Group PC in New York, where she has focused on arbitration and employment law since 2012. "I primarily represent individuals who have faced unlawful treatment in the workplace. The cases range from subtle discrimination to shockingly obvious things you cannot believe still occur. Each case brings its own unique challenges and opportunities to fight for our client."

While "women experiencing menopause" is not itself a protected class, and the case law on discrimination based on menopause is currently limited, Weiner confirmed: "Situations where a woman's menopause symptoms lead to negative treatment due to her age or sex could present legal challenges. I can easily foresee scenarios where women experiencing symptoms may face discrimination in the workplace. Symptoms might impact her performance, potentially leading to unfair treatment due directly to those symptoms."

Symptoms can definitely be disruptive to a woman's work performance. In a 2022 report from Elektra Health based on a survey of 2,000 women ages 40 to 55, 38 percent of women reported missing at least one day of work due to menopause symptoms in the prior year, with 18 percent missing more than four days of work.[186] In addition to hot flashes, the Elektra report found that common menopause symptoms experienced in the workplace by women include fatigue, mood changes, anxiety, weight gain, irritability, headaches, muscle or joint pain, and depression. The majority of women surveyed reported menopause support is lacking relative to other benefits like those for reproductive health or fertility and that they were concerned about cost and affordability of symptom management. Many women, especially women of color, were concerned about ageism if they spoke openly about their symptoms, and chose not to pursue a promotion because of those symptoms.

From a groundbreaking partnership between The Menopause Foundation and Bank of America (BoA), a 2023 survey of two thousand women ages 40 to 65 revealed that more than half of women did not want to discuss menopause at their jobs due to its personal nature, but half of women said menopause negatively affected their work life, because of symptoms like loss of sleep and impacts on physical and/or mental health.[187] Meanwhile, a 2023 survey of more than eight thousand women globally found that nearly half (47 percent) of "women found their work performance disrupted by perimenopause- and menopause-related symptoms"; 40 percent reported six or more different symptoms (including severe symptoms related to sleep or mood) impacting their workplace effectiveness, and 30 percent reported increased stress and decreased concentration and patience at work.[188]

Because women have been taught so little about menopause and how it might affect all areas of life, because it has been treated as a taboo topic in society, and because it has been historically difficult to find a healthcare provider who can actually help, menopause symptoms are generally undertreated and not adequately addressed by traditional healthcare coverage. Accordingly, the (perhaps yearslong) menopause transition can have a profound impact on a woman's daily life, including her work life.

I can guess what you're thinking. *But ... it feels like I just got back from my hard-fought parental leave.* Or: *My employer barely knew about breastfeeding accommodations, and now I'll have to grapple with ones I'll need for menopause?* Or: *I feel like I'm at the point in my career where I'm hitting my stride, finally breaking through the old boys' club. Will menopause stand in my way?* Or: *I took a career pause to take care of my kids and was hoping to get back into paid work now that they're a bit older; is it going to be too hard if I'm also dealing with menopause?* Or any combination of these concerns.

I get it. It does sound like menopause will bring another load of bullshit to a woman's professional success, which is not what we asked for and feels totally unfair.

But if you know me by now, you know I'm an optimist. My friends describe my energy as pink and sparkly, and I hope you get that vibe. So here I will repeat my mother's advice that we first heard in Chapter 3: "If you don't ask, you won't get."

HOW CAN MILLENNIALS PREPARE?

Ask for and Access Benefits

Similar to supportive workplace policies for caregivers, menopause benefits can be logistical (like cooling rooms or access to remote work), cultural (like support groups or informational sessions on the topic), or financial (like spending accounts for menopause products or services or insurance-covered MHT). Such benefits are clearly coveted by working women. The BoA report found that nearly two-thirds of women want some kind of menopause-related benefit.[189] And per the Maven Clinic, millennial women are increasingly indicating that they're more likely to stay at jobs with menopause benefits.[190]

Yet, according to a 2023 Mercer survey, only 15 percent of large organizations (with 500 or more employees) offer or plan to offer specialized menopause benefits like these.[191] While this number is higher than it was a few years ago, it's not nearly high enough. A 2024 Oova survey found that 89.4 percent of women said their work benefits do not cover what they need regarding support for perimenopause (indicating yet again that traditional healthcare does not include care for menopause).[192]

How do we resolve this disconnect? Well, that aforementioned Bank of America survey reported that the number one reason employers don't offer menopause-related benefits is because employees haven't asked for them. So, ask!

Ask now so that you don't wait until you actually need them, when the need will feel urgent and overwhelming. Encourage colleagues—including those decades younger, older, or male—to ask along with you. I'll never forget the group of colleagues I had at a law firm many years ago who helped me advocate for a more comprehensive parental leave policy: women who were older, women who were intentionally child-free, women who were not yet moms, men who were dads, men who weren't, and many others all contributed information, strategy, and support. We successfully got the policy changed, and we did it together. (Thanks again, guys! I think of you often and appreciate you!) It's frustrating, absolutely, that we even have to ask for basic and obviously beneficial things like paid parental leave and menopause-related healthcare—but here we are, so let's ask, together.

Normalize the Need for Menopause-Related Benefits

I frequently hear from older women about how awkward they were made to feel when needing to pump at work before lactation rooms were mandated (and in turn, the need for them was less stigmatized). Just like now we—rightfully—expect our workplaces to provide adequate spaces for nursing mothers and free period products in the bathrooms, we must demand they provide help during the menopause phase of women's lives. Such was emphasized in a 2002 study on menopause education of women in their 20s and 30s, wherein millennial participants expressed sentiments like: "'I think the workplace has a strong need to talk more and educate more on this,' [and] 'Employers should have better understanding. So that it becomes less taboo or something to hide or feel ashamed of.'"[193]

Elektra's cofounder and CEO, a self-identified older millennial and perimenopausal woman of color, Jannine Versi, confirmed to me: "Many employees appreciate access to clinical care related to menopause—but first, they really want education. They want to know what to expect, what the current research is showing, and what trustworthy resources are available." Fortunately, an educational training is a rather simple offering to implement and yet clearly very significant.

If you are an employee, try not to be afraid to talk about why menopause is important to you. It is, after all, important to all women and the people who know them. And if you are an employer reading this, please take note. Destigmatization through education is key! Women are hungry for information and expect and would appreciate it from their place of work.

Request Specific Menopause-Related Trainings and Other Benefits

Ideally the education—and ultimately, the benefits—offered would include information about hormonal approaches as well as nonhormonal treatments so that employees learn about all of their options. The best benefits would also include nutrition and therapeutic support, available through support groups and counseling from specialists.

Millennials believe that mental health matters, including in the workplace. A 2024 survey by workplace benefits company Carrot Fertility found that 75 percent of millennials believe managing menopause symptoms at work will be a moderate or serious challenge, with 56 percent believing menopause will impact their careers; their top concerns (after physical changes and symptoms) are related to mental health and emotional impact.[194] The women surveyed in the Elektra report echoed such concerns: More than two-thirds were worried about how menopause might affect mental health, and 42 percent reported a lack of support (whether emotional or mental health-related) with menopause.[195]

With Americans largely dependent on employers for health insurance, it's imperative that healthcare benefits are comprehensive and not cost-prohibitive, covering all kinds of counseling that may be needed to help women thrive during the menopause transition. Robyn Grosshandler, my breast cancer survivor friend, emphasized the significance of workplaces offering financial support for menopause treatment, including for services that support mental health. She said, "Employees should not feel like they have limited choices on what they can afford when it comes to their quality of life."

Emphasize the Benefits of Menopause Benefits to Employers, Too

If employers don't get with the times when it comes to menopause benefits, employees will likely get going. "If a company doesn't care about its female employees during this major life phase, it's not the kind of company where I'd want to work" is the general theme among most women I know. The millennials surveyed by Carrot agreed; significantly, 70 percent expressed they would consider shifting their work arrangements somehow (perhaps by reducing hours, changing jobs, or retiring early) to mitigate menopause symptoms.[196] Nearly all of the women in the Carrot report (97 percent of millennials; 95 percent of Gen X) said that failing to provide menopause support for employees would be harmful for employers and lead them to lose talent.[197]

"It is definitely in the best interest of employers to support menopause-related issues," Susan Frankel, the healthcare attorney, encouraged. She knows of one international law firm that recently started offering menopause trainings for all employees (Brava!). "Companies have been working on getting women in the boardroom," observed Dr. Brittany Barreto, the FemTech expert. "And now they have to work on keeping them there, by providing women with the right kind of menopause support."

Indeed, as put by an article in *The New York Times* in August 2023, menopause benefits are "the next frontier for corporate benefits," with employers like healthcare company Sanofi and telehealth company Peppy offering such services.[198] When I initially read this, I couldn't help but notice that these two companies were not US-founded. I then learned about the United Kingdom's "Menopause Workplace Pledge" launched by the charity Wellbeing of Women in 2022 to encourage workplaces to be more supportive of this life transition by offering benefits like menopause leave or educational conversations. There are currently more than 3,200 employers signed on, including large institutions like BBC, Tesco, and Royal Mail.[199] I lived in London for two years about a decade ago and frankly felt a bit sorry for myself that I no longer do.

I couldn't help but wonder… Just like paid parental leave, are menopause benefits something Americans will have to fight especially hard for? Maybe.

But maybe not. Happily, by October 2023, several big US-founded companies, including Microsoft Corp., Palantir Technologies Inc., and Abercrombie & Fitch Co., were "among a small but increasing number of US businesses offering menopause benefits," according to a report in *Bloomberg*.[200] By September 2024, more companies like Standard Chartered Plc and Yelp Inc. had been added to the list of those offering benefits like expert-led group sessions or educational content on perimenopause and menopause.[201] I've since learned that additional companies like Genentech[202] and Adobe[203] now offer menopause benefits. Programs like those offered through the Menopause Education Center are now available for menopause in the workplace trainings, and MiDOViA offers menopause-friendly accreditation for US-based companies.

Per a 2024 report by the healthcare platform Maven, companies who rank menopause support as a top priority tend to be large (1,001-10,000 employees) and in the retail and hospitality, professional services, or education industries.[204] Maven's menopause program was its fastest selling, with more than 150 companies signing up within the first nine months of availability.[205] Let's keep adding to the list of employers who provide these kinds of benefits!

I really appreciate that employers seem to be increasingly recognizing their duty to do something about menopause. In a survey of five hundred human resource benefit decision-makers from companies with at least a thousand employees, employers responded that addressing menopause in the workplace was a responsibility shared equally between employee and employer. I firmly believe that the employers that don't address menopause through benefits or otherwise are on the wrong side of history. While it may be on the employee to bring up the subject initially and advocate for what they may need, it's up to the employer to listen, learn, and implement change, or even proactively do so.

And everyone will benefit in the long-term accordingly. Companies that provide menopause support will almost undoubtedly attract and retain talent. The BoA report suggested that women would feel more supported by and connected to the company if such benefits were available, and that employers would expect to see improvement in employee loyalty, productivity, engagement, and other factors.[206]

Menopause isn't something to be ashamed of, yet undoubtedly its effects can feel burdensome to those experiencing it. Women worry about navigating this journey and often feel lonely in doing so. Everyone should remember that this is a natural part of life that is to be expected for half the population. I hope employers continue to recognize the importance of supporting women in midlife.

Cultivate a Kind and Considerate Workplace Culture

There are also some basic things workplaces can provide to women navigating menopause, including flexibility and autonomy (women need time to be able to work out, for example; trust that your employee, an adult, can leave her desk for 25 minutes of much-needed strength training while planning around a nonurgent deadline) or temperature control to help with hot flashes.[207]

Additionally, women are looking for empathy, which is desperately desired in the workplace for a variety of issues including health and caregiving (including self-care). The majority of more than a thousand working women surveyed in 2022 asked for kindness and empathy surrounding menopause.[208] Be the change you wish to see; if someone is having a menopause moment with brain fog or a hot flash, treat them with patience and compassion. One day, for one reason or another, you'll want such an attitude in return.

Empathy is much needed—but also not enough. Acknowledging that menopause deserves support is a good first step, but it's just that. What women also need is access to well-versed professionals who can help them through their symptoms. And workplaces can help with such access through employee healthcare programs, flexible work schedules that allow time for appointments and actual self-care activities, and ensuring that women are not treated differently (i.e., worse) for their menopause-related needs.

If you can't appeal to your employer's humanity, try to appeal to common sense in the form of dollars and cents. As referenced above, without menopause support, women (including talented women who are integral to companies' success) are likely to drop out of the workforce. In addition to impacting them as individuals, this phenomenon would impact women's ability to gain financial security and economic parity with men, cause employers to lose talent and spend money replacing talent, and affect the larger economy. In 2023, The Mayo Clinic estimated that "the total economic burden associated with menopause symptoms is conservatively [!] $26 billion annually in the United States alone."[209]

So please, advocate for expanded menopause-related policies and benefits from your workplace. Advocate even if you're years away from menopause or experienced it years ago. Advocate for it to help other women. I know it's tiring and intimidating on top of all the other things you are dealing with—but if you don't ask, you won't get!

I'm thrilled to share that there are now many free resources available to help you advocate for what you deserve. You can start by using

Bank of America's "Checklist to Help Women Navigate Their Menopause Journey," which includes great tips on having conversations with your employer.[210] You can also pull from or provide Maven's 2024 guide, "Beyond HRT: Building Better Menopause and Midlife Health Benefits,"[211] which points out that men should also receive midlife health support (and, I would emphasize, education on how to support female colleagues and loved ones during menopause) and that companies may provide flexible schedule or menopause leave policies in order to truly support their employees during this phase of life.

The European Menopause and Andropause Society also offers wonderful free resources, including helpful infographics on how employers, organizations, managers, supervisors, and employees with menopause symptoms can implement best practices around menopause in the workplace, including by simply creating an open, inclusive, and supportive culture.[212] In September 2024, The Menopause Society launched its Making Menopause Work initiative with resources including frequently asked questions, sample talking points, employer guides, and various fact sheets and other tools.[213]

While you are advocating for much-needed change in this area, please don't stand for discrimination. It remains a very real issue for women at this stage of life (and always). A 2023 *Harvard Business Review* study found that "'impending menopause'" and "'menopause-related issues'" were actual reasons cited for why some women in their 40s or 50s were not hired for roles in the higher education, faith-based nonprofits, law, and healthcare industries.[214] If you do feel like you're getting treated differently or unfairly at work because of your sex, age, and/or menopause symptoms, keep a detailed record, suggests Weiner. She encouraged, "If further information is needed, including on options for recourse, you should consult with a local employment attorney in your city or state."

I've said it before and I'll say it again: We women (and our allies) must fight back against the deeply ingrained compulsion to be quiet and start talking about these issues, whether outright or subtle discrimination, to create change. In 2024, Sallie Krawcheck, the CEO and founder of Ellevest (an investment platform and financial literacy program for women), wrote about the silence surrounding menopause: "Women have been conditioned to struggle silently, to tough it out, to hold it together. And society, including the workplace, has been conditioned to be complicit in it."[215]

It appears we may be poised for change. That same year, Professor Michelle Travis, codirector of USF's Work Law and Justice Program, wrote about the growing movement to destigmatize menopause in the US for *Forbes*, noting that "women have been increasingly willing to raise legal challenges to menopause discrimination and lack of accommodations in the workplace. Employers can no longer ignore this critical barrier to women's workplace equality."[216]

I hope she's right. I hope that for all women's sake, a more empathetic and supportive workplace is coming. I hope that for millennials' sake, change is coming. Because menopause sure is.

Chapter 12

MILLENNIAL MEN AND MENOPAUSE

• • • • • • • • • • • • • • •

Hey ladies! You didn't think I would leave men out of this conversation, did you? I won't. Menopause may be a life stage experienced by women, but it still very much impacts men. Those men include your husbands, lovers, brothers, fathers, sons, cousins, colleagues, and friends.

I've always been a girly-girl and a feminist—and I've always gotten along well with guys. My good guy friends have been privy to my personal life throughout my life. The first time I purchased condoms at a drugstore was with a male friend. When I had to take Plan B because one of those condoms broke and I felt nauseated at school, a different male friend brought me crackers and listened without judgment. Several male friends served as my "bridesmen"; they threw me a bachelorette party–style dinner prior to and then walked down the aisle during my wedding. The wonderful man I married, in fact, was originally one of my guy friends!

I share this to emphasize that men are very capable of providing emotional support to women when they need it most, like when they are experiencing a life transition. Women sharing wisdom to support each other is incredibly important, yes (!!), but men must also be involved. If we don't include them in reproductive health education, in teaching them about our needs, we risk perpetuating inaccurate gender stereotypes, missing out on meaningful allyship, and contributing to harmful learned helplessness.

Women are not born with the instinctive ability to change a baby's diaper. Instead, they learn how to do it—often sooner than men because they have more opportunities to practice due to cultural expectations including gendered leave policies. But men can and should learn, too. Similarly, women will learn about how menopause may impact their health and other areas of their life because, ultimately, they have to. But I believe men can and should learn, too.

I recognize that they may not need to know all the details. I also see there is an argument to be made for women to learn more about men's health, too (I admittedly know very little about the prostate, for example). And, sure, I'm willing to learn! If the men in your life would say the same, and I hope they would, please hand over this book for a bit. And I'm not just talking about the men you may be in sexual relationships with, but any man in your life who is close to you and wants the best for you.

This chapter is a perimenopause primer for millennial males, a list of Dos and Don'ts for best practices based on advice I've gathered from some of the incredible women I interviewed for this book, and the reflections I have made.

This one's for the boys.

DOS AND DON'TS

Don't Assume You Are Not Relevant to This Conversation

When I set out to write this book, I sent a message to millennial friends and colleagues inquiring what they'd want to learn regarding menopause. One of the aforementioned male friends I've known since before puberty replied: "Good for you Tetty! But as a guy, I don't think I have anything to contribute here."

I responded that his feeling disconnected from even the concept of menopause was exactly the point—as a man born in 1985 with an older sister, a millennial wife, and many other millennial females in his life, he very much has something to contribute here, even if only in question form. What did he want to know about menopause? It turned out he had a lot of thoughtful questions, which I appreciated (and hope to have answered throughout this book). His questions confirmed that our generation is in the dark about this stage of life, even though it is upon us. Men deserve to be informed. To best support women, they need to be informed. Come chat!

And keep talking. It helps normalize this very normal life stage, including for the next generation. My friend Kyle went through surgically induced menopause at 34 and has used a transdermal patch to receive hormone therapy for years. "My boys see me changing my patch and know it's just a part of my personal routine, like changing my contacts," she said of her two young sons. "We all laugh when they make comments like, 'Mommy, you're so hot!' It's all good," she described, and it should be.

Do Educate Yourself Before You Think You Need to Know

"Menopause? Doesn't that start at 70?" the 1983-born husband of a friend of mine asked when he heard about this book. No, sir, it does not. But I understand why he (and maybe you) thought it occurs much later than it actually does at the average age of about 51—because we don't talk about it enough! As a culture we tend to associate menopause with old ladies, and not that there's anything wrong with old ladies, but most millennial men I know wouldn't put a woman in her 40s or 50s in that category. Menopause refers to a woman's next phase of life and reproductive health. It's the end of her fertility, but it is not the end of the world.

Perimenopause is the term we use to describe the phase around menopause, and it can involve several years of physical and emotional symptoms. Women are becoming increasingly educated about perimenopause and think men should be, too. A study published in 2022 about menopause knowledge and education in women under 40 reflected that women "felt it was essential that men were educated on [menopause] too ... the most common feeling was a desire for universal understanding of the menopause so that men become 'less ignorant' and can help support women through this life stage."[217] It's not that you have to become an expert. Simply gaining familiarity with this topic and knowing where to look for more information will ultimately benefit you and your relationships with those you love who are (or eventually will be) menopausal.

As Dr. Rebbecca Hertel, family medicine practitioner and menopause specialist, enthusiastically suggested: "What should men know about menopause? Everything!" At some point, every man will know a woman impacted by menopause—whether that's a mother, a romantic partner, a colleague, or another loved one. Men may not directly experience menopause, but they are certainly affected by it. And by knowing what's going on with the women in their lives, they can help make the experience a better one. "If men understood the impact—both emotional and physical—of menopause on women's lives, it would enable them to be more supportive, empathetic, and understanding," according to Stephanie Falk, cofounder of the mindfulness community Pause to be Present. "It would be a lot less isolating for women if men understood what was happening to the bodies and minds of the women they love during menopause!"

Don't Avoid Talking About It

"Men can help the women in their lives recognize menopause symptoms they may not recognize yet themselves," suggested Dr. Adrienne Mandelberger, gynecologic surgeon and menopause specialist. Common perimenopause symptoms that can easily be dismissed as "just this phase of life" include exhaustion, anxiety, and forgetfulness. But maybe there's more going on, and maybe a woman you know needs a gentle nudge to assess all her symptoms and speak to her healthcare provider about how to handle them.

"Our loved ones can and do observe changes in us," per Susan Frankel, a healthcare attorney whose brothers were incredibly supportive during her menopause transition. "They may need to say, 'You're not yourself. What's going on?' It's invaluable when they are mindful and encouraging." Men can help get a dialogue going and encourage women to speak with professionals about what they are experiencing. They can help validate women's experiences, helping them feel seen, heard, understood, and hopeful, rather than alone.

Do Consider Your Own Health and Lifestyle

Men do not experience a midlife hormonal transition quite the way women do with menopause ("andropause" is the term for the decline in a man's testosterone levels, but very few older men experience levels that are considered low). Still, of course, aging can impact men's health in general. As they age, men may experience changes in their metabolism or physical appearance and become at increased risk of cardiovascular problems, cognitive decline, and certain cancers. Having open conversations about menopause and women's health can help men become more in tune with their own bodies and health needs, and vice versa. Participating in and encouraging healthy habits like regular medical screenings, solid sleep hygiene, and thoughtful diet and exercise routines can go a long way.

Perhaps the biggest difference between men and women at midlife is that fertility for a woman will end at menopause, while a man can produce sperm well into old age. (Think: Al Pacino and Robert De Niro, who each had a baby in 2023, at the age of 83 and 79, respectively.) But don't take this for granted, warned Dr. Lilli Dash Zimmerman, reproductive endocrinologist. "Men must pay attention to their own fertility! About 50 percent of the couples I treat have male infertility. You have to stay on top of these things, especially if you want to grow your family."

Don't Be a Dickhead

Enough with the crude jokes about crazy women and their hormones. Whether you are making them, sharing them, or laughing at them—check yourself. Are you being a nice guy? Would your mother be proud of how you're acting? Remember, a scrub is a guy who won't get no love so don't be one.

The truth is, a perimenopausal woman in your life may be acting different from the woman you know her to be. She may seem moodier, more difficult to appease, and I won't underestimate the toll that can take on you or your relationship. I'm also not suggesting you do nothing about it. But whatever you do, do it with compassion. She is likely not enjoying her symptoms, either!

"Men should know that a menopausal woman's potential mood and weight changes are not signs of character flaws, but rather manifestations of wildly fluctuating hormones," encouraged Dr. Caroline Messer, endocrinologist. There's also a lot going on at midlife (changes in career, family dynamics, general health) that can contribute to stress. About one-third of US adults getting divorced are aged 50 or older,[218] and studies show that women often blame menopause for the breakdown of or strain in their marriage.[219] But it doesn't have to be this way, especially if you approach this new chapter with empathy and understanding.

Some women have told me they feel trapped in their own emotions, with the awareness that they're not quite being rational but feel incapable of calming down the rage or moodiness that rises like a tidal wave. "I feel like I just need to feel my raw emotions, let them out, and then move on without worrying I'm offending my husband, because I know I'm not making complete sense," I've heard.

Cognitive behavioral therapy can help with this, for both of you, as you identify triggers to emotional elevations, responses based on cognitive distortions, and more effective coping mechanisms. Try not to react in a way that adds to her mental load such that she feels she has to take care of you on top of or instead of taking care of herself. This does not mean she can be cruel to you, certainly, but it does mean that together you can develop ways to bring levity or establish boundaries you each need.

Do Take an Active Role in Navigating the Mental Load of Her New Life Chapter*

My guy, millennial women are pretty tired, and I'm not just talking about those in perimenopause. They're not only *doing* a lot at work

---

* After an open discussion with her, of course!

and at home, but they're also *thinking* about doing a lot, which is a heavy burden to bear.

And it's not because they want to take on this mental load or the invisible, unpaid, underappreciated labor—trust me. Rather, they're conditioned and expected to. In the workplace, women are (still!) disproportionately asked to engage in nonpromotable tasks like organizing a holiday party or taking meeting notes, which can detract from career advancement. In the home, women do more caretaking and domestic work, even if they out-earn their male partners, and the cognitive labor involved in this work is associated with women's stress and negative impacts on their mental health and relationships.[220]

Menopause will likely include lots of questions, research, and time spent thinking about its implications and searching for solutions. Help her out. Make her feel like she's not navigating this life transition alone.

It's not quite the same, but consider, if applicable, when the woman in your life was pregnant and/or experiencing fertility issues. She probably went to doctors' appointments without you. She probably engaged in countless hours of research, ranging from perusing social media groups on the "best" baby blankets to interviewing clinicians who would care for your shared child's health. I'm not blaming you for not doing more, because maybe you very well couldn't. My own husband has said of both our kids' births that he struggled with how little he could contribute; he hated feeling helpless.

But I am encouraging you to do more now. Menopause is something that is happening to her, not you, but you are in her life and can help her get through it. Research has shown that men's awareness of menopause and available treatment options can influence their female partners' decisions related to symptom management.[221] "My husband was the one who noticed the changes in my mood and health and attributed it to perimenopause," recalled Fiona Jalinoos, a certified yoga therapist who specializes in supporting women through the menopause transition. "We now very openly discuss menopause issues in our family, and I'm grateful that he has been a true partner."

Consider all the ways you can be a partner. Go to appointments with her healthcare providers, if she wants you to (pro tip: offer before she feels like she has to ask, and don't be offended if she says no). Learn about all the symptom treatment options. Read this entire book!

"It's natural to feel worried about the perimenopause symptoms a woman in your life is experiencing or concerned about the greater health implications," confirmed Kara Cruz, licensed marriage and family therapist. "Together, you can gain knowledge. You can help her carry some of the emotional weight."

Don't Take a Low Sex Drive Personally

It's not you, it's her. Probably. (Disclaimer: This is not a guarantee. Either way, talk to her!)

Women in perimenopause may not be sleeping well, may not be loving their midlife bodies, may be experiencing vaginal pain, and may be feeling sad, anxious, or otherwise just not in the mood. A low libido is not ideal, I know, for her, either. And we should not forget that you likewise may be experiencing changes to your mood, body, or libido due to hormone changes (specifically, the loss of testosterone) common for men at midlife.

Please do not be offended or reactive if the woman in your life isn't feeling much of a sex life lately. Instead, ask her how she's doing. Ask her if there is anything you can do. Check in with her as to whether sex is feeling painful, which is a common symptom for midlife women. "Open communication is incredibly important," advised Melissa Ferrara, family nurse practitioner and women's sexual health expert.

Ferrara also encourages women and their partners to manage their expectations around sex, even when treatment to improve libido is implemented. For example, Addyi, the prescription drug available to treat hyposexual dysfunction disorder in premenopausal women (Have you heard of it? It seems most women haven't, so feel free to spread the word), should be used for at least two to three months to see if it's working, and "working" can mean different things to different people. "Medications are not always a slam dunk, and not for all women. The benefits may be subtle. But that may still be a great improvement for some women," Ferrara clarified.

In addition to or in the alternative of medication that can influence sex drive, she suggests women and their partners consider behavioral modifications like reading or watching or listening to erotica ("Together or solo—the brain is one of the biggest sex organs there is, and it's important women get comfortable with fantasizing!") and learning how to connect again ("Hold hands, cuddle, have intimacy without sexual intercourse so you can feel reconnected."). Ferrara also explained that while it doesn't sound sexy, scheduling sex brings about relief and removes feelings of potential rejection. Sex therapist Dr. Carli Blau also regularly encourages this. "Think of how you scheduled intimacy—physical or emotional—while first dating and scheduling time to meet up," she put into perspective.

Do Offer Support in Whatever Way It's Needed

I think (hope) that millennial men are going to be supportive about menopause. "I see a shift in your generation around parenting and gender roles," observed Deborah Duke, a registered nurse who was born in 1949. "I think it's shifting for the better. I think men today have a more caring mindset."

Guys, I know you care. One of you even wrote me about millennials and menopause: "What should I be doing as a husband?" This is exactly the kind of question you should be asking! I can't advise on every situation, but I think I can say generally, that you can—and should—simply check in on how you can be supportive. One of the most important factors in any relationship is open communication, and that applies to biological transitions like menopause, too.

And then of course, listen to—really pay attention to—the answer.

"When women are supported, the menopausal transition is much easier than when they are not," confirmed Dr. Kathy Casey, an acupuncture and Eastern medicine provider. And support comes in all kinds of forms. You can be supportive as a man who advocates for menopause benefits in the workplace. You can be supportive as a man who teaches his kids, whatever their gender, about respecting women's bodies and about the need to destigmatize issues related to women's sexuality and health. You can be supportive as a man who researches symptoms and treatment options or who funds or demands research on a broader level.

You can also be a friend, family member, or partner who shows he cares through simple gestures. My family friend Karen, who went through menopause about 30 years ago, shares a funny story about her hot flashes: "I hadn't slept in months. I was so uncomfortable throughout the night, and I was so, so exhausted. Then suddenly one night, I figured out the right pajamas to wear and the right thermostat situation. I finally slept. My husband noticed; the next morning, he told me he was glad I got a good night's sleep. I looked over at him while he said so and realized he was wearing two sweatshirts and the thermal pants he usually wore skiing. 'I was about to break out my earmuffs,' he said, laughing about how cold it was in our bedroom. But he said he'd have been happy to, and I believed him, which meant the world to me."

Before you whip out your winter gear (which is an easy and adorable way to show you care, I agree), try something even simpler: Ask her how you can be supportive. Seriously, just go ask.

You'll thank me later. And I thank you for reading.

Chapter 13

GIRL POWER

Where my girls at? Now that we've had our chat with the guys, let's check back in, ladies.

Women are becoming increasingly active about menopause, and I love to see it.

In many ways, celebrities have been at the center of this cultural conversation. They have participated in if not led numerous projects and initiatives about menopause throughout 2024, and I expect more to come. I am so grateful to them for using their platforms to help other women. Stars, they're just like us!

Thank you, Halle Berry, for advocating in front of Congress in May 2024 to pass bipartisan legislation to invest in menopause-related healthcare and research.* Thank you, Alyssa Milano, for producing a docuseries about perimenopause. Thank you, Naomi Watts, for all you've done to raise awareness and lower stigma about this natural life stage, including launching your pro-aging beauty brand, Stripes, and writing your book about beginning perimenopause at 36. Thank you, Whoopi Goldberg, for your graphic novel about a woman embracing superpowers gained through menopause. Thank you, Kate Winslet, for speaking on podcasts about how testosterone hormone therapy can help women's libido. Thank you, *One Tree Hill* star and millennial celeb Hilarie Burton for openly talking about periods and perimenopause in various settings.

Thank you, Michelle Obama, Drew Barrymore, Oprah Winfrey, and many other famous women for speaking up about these issues, for helping normalize them, and for offering resources we desperately need. America loves celebrities, so if they are what it takes to help women be heard, then by all means, keep speaking up!

It seems it's not just Hollywood that's having a menopause moment, but also Wall Street (perhaps too little too late, but we'll take it).

The global menopause market in 2023 was estimated to be worth $16.93 billion, with expected growth of its market size value to reach $24.4 billion by 2030.[222] It's projected to continue to grow to $27.6 billion by 2033.[223] Since these figures cover only menopause-related dietary supplements and over-the-counter pharmaceutical options (both hormonal and nonhormonal), they are likely underestimates; the market for all menopause products and services is much bigger.[224]

---

* The aforementioned H.R. 6749—Menopause Research and Equity Act of 2023.

"The numbers are really all over the place at the moment," observed Pooja Rajput, a millennial and a managing director of healthcare services at a global financial institution. "We are in such nascent stages of research related to menopause, and I think that business opportunity really follows the research. There are currently lots of exciting opportunities in this space."

Dr. Brittany Barreto agreed: "In the last five years we've seen a lot of activity in the menopause market, including the founding of 75 percent of the companies currently out there. There are many good options for telehealth and hormone therapy offerings, and we're also seeing growth in areas to help manage symptoms like hot flashes, brain fog, and vaginal dryness." About $244 million has been invested in the menopause industry so far, and approximately 40.4 percent of that has been allocated to consumer-packaged goods companies.[225] The products offered range from tracking bracelets to bedding items like cooling blankets to red light therapies. "The market is not yet oversaturated," per Dr. Barreto, "because the issue is not yet solved." So keep 'em coming!

Some research has indicated that the menopause space represents $600 billion of spending opportunity.[226] A recent AARP survey found that women spend over $13 billion each year on treating menopause symptoms, including more than $2.7 billion on menopausal hormone therapy, more than $10 billion on nonmedical treatments like supplements or other wellness practices, and more than $4.5 million on copays for treatments and services somewhat covered by their insurance plans.[227] Another study found that the average woman spends $2,000 per year on products and services related to menopause over a 10-year period (that's an average of $20,000 total for fellow nonmath folks).[228] Plus, consider the unquantifiable but very significant mental, logistical, and emotional costs of searching for helpful treatments, perhaps while you are really struggling, over the course of several years!

We've already learned a bit about the innovative start-ups in this space, including Alloy, Elektra, and Midi, that provide virtual care and community in addition to supplements and pharmaceutical products. There's clearly a lot of money to be spent—and made—on menopausal care products and services. You would think they'd get financial support from tons of investors who see their obvious value to the billions of women around the world experiencing menopause symptoms, right?

Not exactly, sorry to say—but perhaps you are not shocked, since we've already talked about how it seems like this issue receives too little care.

Research reflects that only 7 percent of FemTech companies concentrate on menopause care,[229] and that menopause companies receive only about 3 to 5 percent of venture capital funding.[230] Experts tend to believe that the lack of investment is due to the usual: sexism, ageism, and a discomfort with menopause in general. "Since the space is led by predominantly female founders, they are facing challenges to raise capital from male investors who have no understanding of the condition,'" per Dr. Barreto.[231] She and researcher Ludovica Castiglia have found women's health tech companies—meaning, to be clear, companies that are designed *for women* and their health issues—are less likely to get funding if a woman is on the founding team, particularly when potential investors perceive her passion for the purpose is greater than that for profits.[232]

"It's a real issue that menopause is not getting the attention nor financial backing it deserves," noted Rajput. "Nearly all of the pitches I've seen are from women, which may be OK because it's hard to understand a need until you actually feel the need. But the larger concern is the investor base, which is mostly men. They don't connect with the founders and consider menopause a 'niche' issue. But it's not. It's mainstream."

Case in point: When Elektra Health was launched in 2019, cofounder and CEO Jannine Versi recalled that it took a lot of time to educate investors on why they should care about the issue of menopause. "But now investors do seem to recognize that they are missing out if they haven't bought into this issue yet. Other healthcare issues, like fertility—which is incredibly important but affects only about 12 percent of the population—are not nearly as wide-ranging in their impact. About 50 percent of the population will be affected one way or another by menopause." Another way of thinking about it is, not every woman wants to or will be a parent, but every woman will experience menopause. Versi explained, "It struck me that a lot of FemTech companies were focused on a woman's reproductive years. But what happens when you're past that?"

Anne Fulenwider shared that Alloy has been fairly fortunate when it comes to financial support; in November 2024, the startup raised $16 million from investors. When the company first started, though, reactions were "all over the map. I do think there is some bias because menopause—aging, especially women aging—is not sexy." However, the numbers don't lie. As she argued, "Half the population will undergo this universal experience, and about 80 percent of women will have moderate symptoms and are looking for answers." It's not an exaggeration to say that this is a big, *big* market.

Fortunately, Rajput reported, investment trends are changing. "I am now seeing more men team up with women at these pitches. That's a welcome sight, but we still have a long way to go."

HOW CAN MILLENNIALS PREPARE?

Tell Your Story

Use your power to tell your story, whether you are a celebrity or a layperson. It not only helps with alleviating isolation but also with accessing investments. "We've seen a direct correlation between funding for certain health conditions and media coverage," revealed Dr. Barreto. "We've done studies with investors, discovering that if they hadn't heard of an issue, they assumed it was niche and there was no money to be made. But, once they heard about it multiple times in mainstream media, they felt like it was a real thing deserving of innovation."

We all know that menopause isn't niche, and yet it has not gotten the media coverage it deserves. Until—maybe, hopefully—now.

Put Your Money Where Your Mouth Is

We should all invest in women and women's issues, friends. The future is female. At the very least, about half our global population is. "Why should we invest in menopause healthcare? Why *wouldn't* we?" prompted Rajput. "It makes business sense as much as quality-of-life sense. We need diversity at senior levels so we can continue to create awareness and actually find supportive solutions."

Because menopause is such an individualized experience that affects such a large number of people, there are various ways to make an impact. As Versi said, "There is room for everyone in the menopause space. There is not one single organization or doctor that will dominate it or is doing things the right way." Fulenwider agreed: "We have 70 million women looking for solutions. The more providers and companies focused on this problem, the better. Women deserve access and support."

While our sisters are making strides in the media and with money when it comes to menopause, women must be cautious about what they are consuming to alleviate their symptoms. "There's an overwhelming amount of information out there on social media and predatory marketing toward menopausal women[233] to purchase things like miracle creams, making them feel further lost during this transition," observed Dr. Leah Ansell, the dermatologist. She and I both believe that we need products and services based in science and offered as part of individualized care for each woman. That's why it's so important to find a medical provider who is informed about peri/menopause, and whom you really trust to listen and take your issues seriously.

Empower Each Other to Achieve Change

Women may be able to finally get what we deserve if we advocate for a more integrative healthcare approach. Research reflects that medical care in a group setting may be a useful option for midlife women in order to improve their access to evidence-based, comprehensive care.[234] Trained, licensed, or certified menopause doulas or coaches are also increasingly available and popular among women who feel their needs have not been met by traditional healthcare providers.[235]

"Ideally, women going through menopause should be treated by a multidisciplinary team," suggested Dr. Shieva Ghofrany, the OB/GYN and cancer survivor. "All the practitioners should collaborate, and insurance should cover the visits and cover them well. Women deserve coordinated care!"

Of course, for some women this isn't readily possible given the price of healthcare and the complexity of the system in the United States. To truly benefit all women, we must also advocate for better policies. We can use our power to vote for elected officials who can enact legislation that actually benefits us. If any type of healthcare reform is important to you, try focusing on your county and state elections, do your research, and show up to vote in *every* election. You may consider volunteering for the campaigns or candidates who will bring about the type of change you want to see most. We've seen this be effective in certain countries and jurisdictions.

In England, for example, residents who have a prescription for eligible hormone replacement therapy medicine can get a "prescription prepayment certificate" from the United Kingdom's publicly funded healthcare system, the National Health Service (NHS), that will cover all eligible medications for 12 months at the cost of £19.80 (approximately $25.60), which is basically the cost of two single prescription charges.* Millions of women have taken advantage of this program since it was implemented in 2023[236] due to the advocacy of Member of Parliament Carolyn Harris, an elected official committed to ensuring that women will no longer need to silently endure menopause.[237] In 2024, British Columbia, along with the federal government, became the first Canadian province to help finance hormone replacement therapy. The country's Federal Health Minister indicated that doing so is, "fundamentally important for women's health[…] 'And the fact that so many women can't afford that treatment [until now] means fundamentally devastating things for their health.'"[238] Women in Canada also report feeling increasingly more comfortable discussing their menopause-related needs in menopause-friendly work environments.[239] As of January 2025, women in Ireland experiencing menopause symptoms are invited to apply for free hormone replacement therapy products, expected to save between €360 and €840 a year (approximately $386 to $900), due to an amendment to the Health Insurance Bill.[240]

In the United States, as Versi of Elektra told me: "We need to bake menopause care into the fabric of basic healthcare for people. That's where government and public health can step in. This is not an elective or aesthetic issue, but rather fundamental, basic care for 50 percent of the population. Such care must become accessible to women of all races, socioeconomic status, employment status."[241] She explained that Elektra's next phase of growth is to become

---

* Learn more at https://www.gov.uk/get-a-ppc/hrt-ppc.

embedded in healthcare plans, including Medicare and Medicaid. "We are working with stakeholders including health systems to deliver services and make menopause care accessible to all women."

For now, we're seeing growth in private-sector areas like FemTech, per Dr. Barreto.[242] But perhaps soon enough, we won't even need a distinct label. "Shouldn't all healthcare include increasing access to care for half of humanity?" pondered Rajput.

Yes, I believe it should. And I am encouraged by the optimism of the many experts with whom I've spoken. I hope you are, too.

"I do feel like the future of women's health is bright," shared Dr. Barreto. "Think about how much women have accomplished already with so few rights and while not feeling our best. We have opportunities now that we've never had before—we have to use our voice to empower each other!"

Chapter 14

WHAT'S NEXT AFTER WHAT'S NEXT?

Let's remind ourselves that many women who have experienced menopause feel a huge sense of relief. *Bye bye bye to all that period bullshit,* they cheer about the breakup of perhaps their longest companion. *We are never (ever) getting back together!*

While not worrying about menstruating or unwanted pregnancy is certainly worth celebrating, the final menstrual period and the year that follows do not necessarily bring total freedom from menopause symptoms. It wasn't over at your last period and it still isn't over. Sorry to burst that bubble.

"For the majority of women, the ups and downs of perimenopause, including brain fog, emotional symptoms, and the extreme hot flashes, tend to improve or totally resolve once they reach actual menopause or within a few years after," explained Dr. Adrienne Mandelberger. "But in general, there are very important disease states or risk factors, as well as specific symptoms of menopause, that stay or get worse after actual menopause and can last the rest of a woman's life."

And as we've learned, some women do not experience menopause symptoms at all. But their bodies are still changing as they enter into the postmenopause phase, which means that attention to one's health remains paramount. Per Dr. Mandelberger: "Postmenopause, you'll be dealing with risk factors related to cardiovascular health, dementia, etc. You must continue to speak with your healthcare provider about your health, and the 'one size does not fit all' approach still applies."

I won't go into too many details here about all the possible postmenopause symptoms because I think that generally, millennials are still getting their heads around perimenopause and the fact that it is happening much sooner than originally anticipated (i.e., now). But let's take a brief look at some of the common issues that postmenopausal women may have to contend with in life's next chapter. Please note that menopause is not the underlying *cause* of these issues; rather, the menopause transition is linked to increased risks for them, which can severely impact health and quality of life. (Please also keep in mind that this is not an exhaustive list and, as you know, definitely not medical advice!)

GENITOURINARY SYMPTOMS, INCLUDING PAINFUL SEX AND UTIs

Menopause, with its changes in a woman's hormones and to vaginal tissue, can lead to genitourinary symptoms (those that affect the urinary and genital organs). The symptoms can, and are actually likely to, worsen if not treated. The various symptoms are often referred to by the term "genitourinary syndrome of menopause (GSM)," which affects about half of postmenopausal women.[243] Providers use the term "vaginal dyspareunia" for pain that can occur before, during, or after sex, and note that there can be many contributing factors to this condition for postmenopausal women, including vaginal or vulvar atrophy (when there is painful inflammation due to tissue thinning because of low estrogen levels), sexually transmitted infection (which is often underdiagnosed in women at midlife),[244] and pelvic floor problems. (As pelvic floor expert Sara Reardon described: "Your hormones are shot at that point, compounded by the muscle mass decrease that too often goes unaddressed.") Forget what you may have done there one time at band camp—during menopause, you may not even want to go near your vag.

Vaginal dryness is perhaps the most common GSM symptom, affecting up to 93 percent of women.[245] What might that mean in real life? If you're thinking of the classic line from *Heathers* about a chainsaw, you're getting the right idea, unfortunately. "After I went through menopause, my vagina felt like sandpaper," a woman born in 1965 told me. "I could barely sit because of the stinging sensation. It felt like I had a UTI permanently." Ouch!

Speaking of, UTIs themselves can be common, even chronic, for postmenopausal women. This is because the loss in estrogen leads to "dryness, irritation, and other changes that set the stage for UTIs," according to ACOG.[246] Estrogen loss can also weaken the urethra muscles, providing more opportunity for bacteria to enter the urethra and move into the bladder, and often leads to less healthy bacteria to help prevent infections. And if you're lucky to not know what a UTI feels like, imagine feeling like it burns when you pee, and that you have to pee *all the time*.

UTIs are *really* not fun at best, and life-threatening at worst. Dr. Mandelberger noted that many older women misunderstand that some symptoms can worsen after menopause. "I've seen women in their 80s dismiss these kinds of symptoms because they have gotten over other symptoms. But when you're older, your nervous system is not working like it's used to. An untreated UTI can lead to urosepsis and can kill you." Whenever you're feeling like something isn't right, please don't ignore it!

BONE DENSITY LOSS

We've highlighted the importance of eating well and exercising right to maintain bone density throughout your 30s. While it's never too early (or too late) to start, strong bones are particularly important at midlife. Studies show that at age 40, women begin to lose bone at a rate of .3% to .5% per year; during menopause, they experience bone loss at 10 times that rate![247]

Many women in perimenopause experience low back pain that can continue through the menopause transition.[248] I mean, my back hurts right now—admittedly I'm in a turtle-like position at my (hot pink, of course) desk, but this can't bode well for my future.* Per the Endocrine Society, one in two postmenopausal women will have osteoporosis, and most will suffer a broken bone during their lifetime, leading to pain, decreased mobility, and function.[249] Many women suffer hip fractures, leading to increased depressive symptoms, pain, and cost related to adequate long-term care. I'd definitely like to not be one of those women, how about you?

CARDIOVASCULAR DISEASE (CVD)

Did you know that cardiovascular disease kills more women than all forms of cancer combined? It's heartbreaking, literally, that so little attention is paid to this area of health, with women still underrepresented in heart health trials[250] and treated according to guidelines for men if treated at all.[251] Women continue to be underdiagnosed and unaware of their risks of cardiovascular disease. However, CVD is behind 33 percent of deaths in women per year, according to the American Heart Association.[252]

It's not that menopause causes cardiovascular disease, but rather that it causes changes to a woman's bodily functions. Therefore, menopause occurs at a point in midlife when women's CVD risk

---

* Note to reader—and to self—sit up straight! Lisa Schoenholt of Brooklyn Embodied Pilates suggests sitting on top of your sitz bones on the base of your pelvis, with your ribs stacked over your hips. "Think long spine and relaxed shoulders."

factors can also accelerate. But rest assured that there are some options to explore and discuss with your provider at midlife to mitigate your risk.

In particular, estrogen can provide a protective effect against heart disease in women. Numerous healthcare providers told me that estrogen helps lower the level of the "bad kind" of cholesterol (LDL) while maintaining the "good kind" (HDL). Cardiologist and women's heart health expert Dr. Anais Hausvater explained, "When the body endures estrogen withdrawal, the health of the arteries can be affected. Arteries feeding the brain can become stiff, and risk of stroke can be increased. Estrogen also protects against the buildup of plaque, so when it decreases, there is a risk of increased plaque buildup that can lead to a heart attack."

Accordingly, postmenopausal women who have experienced drops in estrogen are at increased risk of cardiovascular disease, including higher cholesterol, blood pressure, and risk of stroke.[253] Black women in particular tend to experience more (and earlier) heart issues.[254] Studies have linked menopausal vasomotor symptoms (hot flashes, night sweats) with heart health issues.[255] While we still don't have enough data on how exactly hot flashes and stroke risk are linked, hot flashes can be clues to women's heart health.

Continuous monitoring of cardiovascular risk factors (such as cholesterol and glucose) is recommended to assess cardiovascular risk among women during the menopause transition. Dr. Hausvater described: "Menopause, like pregnancy-related complications or a history of breast cancer, is a female-specific condition that can enhance cardiovascular disease risk." So it is important to discuss your history and all of these potential risk factors with your healthcare providers. If you haven't been to a primary care physician in many years, consider making an appointment now so you can have some baseline data on hand as you age. Engage in regular health screenings and don't assume symptoms like hot flashes are not potentially serious.

COGNITIVE IMPAIRMENT

As mentioned above, vasomotor symptoms like hot flashes have also been linked to cognitive functioning, with severe menopause symptoms observed among postmenopausal women with mild cognitive impairment.[256] In fact, "accumulating evidence suggests an association between vascular disease and cognitive decline and dementia."[257] In general, per the American Heart Association and other research, risk factors for problems with heart health (including high blood pressure, diabetes, and obesity) increase the likelihood for problems with brain health, including cognitive decline and dementia.[258]

Some background info for you: "Dementia" is an umbrella term for symptoms that affect cognitive function. Dementia diagnoses are on the rise: One person is diagnosed with dementia every seven seconds.[259] Alzheimer's is a specific type of dementia—the most common type—and disproportionately affects women. In fact, about two-thirds of Americans with Alzheimer's are women.[260]

How does menopause fit in? We know that women who naturally or surgically experience premature (before age 40) or early (before age 45) menopause are at higher risk of dementia as well as of cardiovascular disorders, hypertension, weight gain, and midlife diabetes, all of which can also increase the risk of cognitive disorders.[261] But it's inaccurate to say that menopause causes dementia. Remember, correlation is not causation! Instead, it can be thought of as a risk factor. Neuroscientist Dr. Lisa Mosconi, the director of the Alzheimer's Prevention Program and of the Women's Brain Initiative, indicated to *The New York Times* in 2023 that the links between menopause and Alzheimer's are not yet fully understood.[262] She is currently running a clinical trial[263] on the effect of estrogen menopausal hormone therapy on brain metabolism and cognition to test if it has an effect on some of the earliest biomarkers of Alzheimer's.[264] In February 2025, she joined as program director a new $50 million research program established with the goal of preventing millions of Alzheimer's cases in women by focusing on hormones and endocrine aging. But until studies like hers are completed and their data published, we can't say for certain exactly how or why menopause and Alzheimer's may be linked.

In the meantime, Dr. Pauline Maki of the University of Illinois at Chicago, who is an expert on cognitive health and menopause, offered this perspective to *The New York Times*: "Consider how many women go through menopause—every woman, right? And 80 percent of them will not get dementia … We can't catastrophize this universal transition."[265] I agree, though we should be aware of our potential risks. And, as discussed further below, be prepared to mitigate them.

ANXIETY AND DEPRESSION

Not to make light of mental health, but if you're feeling a little anxious or depressed after reading all of these health issues potentially headed your way postmenopause, well, I get it. I understand that it may feel like I just dumped on you a bunch of dreadful health conditions to contend with. Plus, postmenopausal women are grieving their reproductive years, and perhaps children they wanted but now cannot have. They're also experiencing estrogen-related changes to their appearance, including loss of skin firmness and larger pores, making their own reflection in the mirror unrecognizable and creating further dissonance with their own identities.

It seems natural, then, that postmenopausal women often experience mental health symptoms, as well. It is estimated that 20 percent of people aged 55 years or older experience some type of mental health concern like anxiety, depression, or another co-occurring disorder; being a female continues to be a risk factor for mental health issues like depression.[266]

Like other health issues, it's not necessarily that menopause causes anxiety and depression; but rather, it presents an opportunity for increased risk. Menopause can be thought of as a window of opportunity for depression and anxiety because of all the biopsychosocial changes happening at once. Mood disorder symptoms can be exacerbated by life transitions, including loss of a loved one, retirement, or divorce, as well as hormonal and physical changes like menopause and the health issues discussed above. Research reflects that anxiety and depression are more severe in postmenopausal women from rural or low socioeconomic areas.[267]

Bottom line? When women don't get the right kind of support as they navigate major changes, including menopause, their mental health will be negatively impacted.

HOW CAN MILLENNIALS PREPARE?

Keep Talking

In college every Tuesday night our local bar had live music. I used to hop up onstage (oh, youth) and sing "Don't Stop Believin'"—and I'm thinking I may need to modify the lyrics now to "Don't Stop Talkin.'" Because postmenopause, we're not done, even though our periods may be.

"Many older women, especially those who went through menopause under the shadow of the 2002 WHI study that effectively reduced their treatment options, avoid talking about menopause and the related symptoms altogether," observed Dr. Mandelberger. "They'll say things like, 'I don't want to talk about it, I'm through with all that,' reflecting the sort of trauma they've been through regarding their health." But, she warned, postmenopause is best thought of as a new state of your body's being that will last the rest of your life. "It's absolutely worth talking and learning about your symptoms, treatment options, history, risks, and goals, so that you feel as good as possible postmenopause. You deserve it."

Optimize Your Lifestyle Now

And you deserve to optimize your health and lifestyle now, for later, and for the rest of your life. Everything is connected and multilayered, like the fact that good cardiovascular health is linked to improved cognitive outcomes. Let's consider some of the strategies we explored in Chapter 9 in connection with perimenopause and now apply them to postmenopause, including exercise, sleep, self-compassion, and medication.

"A healthy lifestyle now—in terms of nutrition (less alcohol, more protein and fiber), exercise, quality sleep, and stress reduction—will all help with reducing inflammation, which will help with postmenopause symptoms and improve health," Dr. Mandelberger advised. "Younger women should act now to get themselves in the best possible situation going into menopause. A life can be long, but let's focus on health-span vs. lifespan. You can extend life, but really, you want to be healthy! We need to make changes now so that we can prolong our health-span." Your health is your wealth, indeed.

I can't guarantee that movement like walking and weight-bearing exercise will help you avoid postmenopause symptoms altogether, but all the experts I spoke with agree that they would help enhance your health. "Physical fitness and muscle gains—which can be implemented at any age—can help with all chronic diseases associated with aging," confirmed Dr. Mandelberger. "You must build muscle mass, it is so crucial." Building muscle mass through strength training can help boost metabolism and increase bone density. Plus, if you are on any weight loss drugs, building muscle mass makes their effects more sustainable.

Menopause experts often explain that muscle mass building can help with heart health, diabetes risk, brain health, longevity, metabolism, body composition, and balance, including the ability to prevent broken bones upon falling. Anita Mirchandani, the nutritionist and fitness professional, clarified: "Don't worry about calorie burning or lifting super heavy weights. Don't strain yourself if your body can't handle it or do exercises you used to do in your 30s. Figure out movement that suits you at this new phase of life."

Frailty may be increased by menopause, but physical activity programs can help—but only when actually adhered to, which is more likely with social support and interaction. So grab a girlfriend and get going!

I can tell you firsthand that having your betches by your side helps. I am so lucky that two women close to me, Tara Sussman and Jessica Press, teach exercise classes (yoga and dance, respectively) that always remind me there is such joy in moving to fun music with your friends. As I've learned the importance of strength training, I've started working out with two friends (Marisa and Melissa—can't you tell we're '80s babies?!) to help hold me accountable. Aerobic, resistance, and balance exercises have proved effective at increasing bone mineral density in postmenopausal women, but really, there is something for everyone, at every age.[268] Weight-bearing exercises (including lifting weights, running, climbing stairs, hiking, dancing, tennis, and other sports) can help prevent the loss of bone mass, while exercises like Pilates can alleviate menopause symptoms and increase lumbar strength and flexibility for postmenopausal women.[269] You don't need expensive or extensive equipment and can instead use your own body weight and engage in squats, crunches, and push-ups (my least fave but hey, I'm trying!).

As Kelly, Jessie, and Lisa from Bayside High once sang: "Put your mind to it, go for it, get down and break a sweat." Dr. Austin, the sports medicine doctor, advised that it is best practice for women to employ lifestyle changes like strength training exercises as soon as possible. "I think it's important to build up your bone strength naturally, doing anything you can like implementing a healthy diet and exercise routine," she suggested. "If you have to stop MHT for whatever reason—or if you never want to start it—you want to do the work that you can to prevent osteoporosis or stress fractures. Some things *are* in your control!"

Some favorite behaviors can make a positive impact, too: sex and sleep. Sleep continues to affect just about everything else for women at this stage. Poor sleep can impact weight (including menopause belly fat, often referred to as a fat roll) and in turn one's body image, self-esteem, libido, and CVD risk. Additionally, "the risk of developing sleep apnea doubles after menopause," according to Dr. Nishi Bhopal, the sleep psychiatrist, "because of changes in hormones and body weight and the redistribution of fat, which can lead to airway obstruction during sleep." Similar to heart health, sleep issues in women are not studied nearly enough, and we do not recognize them as easily. "Sleep apnea in women can look quite different than it does in men," Dr. Bhopal explained. "While some women may experience classic sleep apnea symptoms like snoring, daytime sleepiness, and gasping for air during sleep, other women may have symptoms that look like insomnia, brain fog, fatigue, chronic pain, or depression."

Research shows that therapeutic massage can improve sleep quality in postmenopausal women.[270] Cognitive behavioral therapy for insomnia can also help with menopausal sleep problems.[271] Per Dr. Bhopal, other interventions that can be helpful in treating both depression and sleep issues, which have a bidirectional relationship (meaning they influence each other, creating a cycle), include maintaining a consistent wake time to regulate the body's circadian rhythm, getting bright sunlight exposure outdoors or via a bright light therapy device within 30 minutes of waking up, eating nutritious meals regularly, and socializing and staying connected with family, friends, and community.

The significance of social connection at midlife should not be underestimated. "Socialize! That is a huge part of brain health, including memory and mood," encouraged Dr. Silverstein, the neurologist. "Socializing keeps us healthy and feeling connected, which is so important for our emotional and mental health." She added that keeping your brain active can include simple activities like reading every day, since reading builds muscle memory and neural connections. "You can also play word games like Scrabble, do puzzles, or watch *Jeopardy*. The earlier you start, the better."

Sex may be part of that social connection for postmenopausal women. Please take to heart that sex should not be painful. Many clinicians report that women essentially try to convince themselves that pain during sex (including self-stimulation) is a natural part of aging. So many women tell themselves it's not a big deal or to just live with it. While some changes can be expected, they are not insurmountable and should not be dismissed. I know it can feel really awkward, but please speak with your doctor about your sexual activity and what isn't feeling quite right, if anything. There could be numerous factors at play and a variety of ways to treat symptoms. Remember, if you don't ask, you won't get.

You know how a few chapters ago we talked about getting your groove back in perimenopause? Well even postmenopause, you could and should still be sexual (if you want to be)! In fact, studies have shown that many women aged 45 and older have at least moderate sexual desire and that the majority of sexually active women aged 50 to 80 are satisfied with their sexual activity.[272] And, sex is not only important for your mental and relationship health, but also your physical health—it can help stimulate blood flow and maintain the vagina's stretchiness.

Collaborate with Healthcare Providers

Women should be informed about the wide range of safe treatment options for any genitourinary symptoms leading to painful sex or general discomfort down there. Diverse treatment options are currently being researched, including laser treatment to improve blood flow in the vaginal tissue, but more data are needed on their effectiveness. Melissa Ferrara, the nurse practitioner who specializes in women's sexual health, suggests behavioral strategies like audio erotica, pelvic floor therapy, vibrators, and sex ed apps and websites. Innovative treatments like the O-Shot offered at Ferrara's clinic, which promotes sensitivity in the vaginal canal intended to help women achieve orgasm, may also be helpful.

And don't forget the proven efficacy of menopausal hormone therapy in its various forms. Remember that vaginal estrogen treatment is safe and effective, even for women who have had hormone receptor-positive cancers or who are on systemic MHT, since the cream specifically targets the vagina.[273] MHT can be helpful beyond GMS symptoms, too. For example, like vaginal estrogen, localized estrogen in the form of a face cream is thought to be safe and can improve the way menopausal women's skin looks and feels by enhancing elasticity; its efficacy is currently being studied by companies like Alloy.[274]

As for menopausal hormone therapy in general, it can be effective (depending on type, form, dosage, point of onset, and other individual factors) to prevent against bone loss, to promote brain health, and to protect against cardiovascular problems.[275] Barring a contraindication, as referenced in Chapter 6, MHT is usually recommended for women who have their ovaries removed before the typical age of spontaneous menopause to help with these issues.[276] In particular, a 2024 study of more than 34,600 women in the UK found that women who experienced early bilateral oophorectomies (i.e., surgically induced menopause) who use hormone therapy and those with increased education have lower odds of developing Alzheimer's disease.[277]

MHT can have other potential benefits, the nuances of which we are seeing in more and more research. For example, a recent study found it helpful with weight loss in conjunction with a semaglutide medication.[278] And though MHT is still not considered a first-line treatment for issues like bone density loss[279] or as a preventative strategy for cognitive decline or cardiovascular issues, more research can be illuminative and can help dispel the misconceptions we're still living with more than 20 years after the 2002 WHI study. As always, women and their healthcare providers should take an individualized approach, including various risk assessments, to menopausal hormone therapy.

And now, you may be wondering on behalf of your future self: *If I do decide to start using menopausal hormone therapy to treat my symptoms, when should I stop?*

"The advice used to be that women should be on the lowest dose of hormones for the shortest amount of time," per Dr. Rebbecca Hertel, the family doctor and menopause specialist. "But now that theory can be considered alarmist, conservative, and no longer the general rule of thumb," she explained, in line with the latest guidance from The Menopause Society.[280] The nurse practitioner and menopause specialist Natalie Givargidze elaborated: "The Menopause Society guidelines no longer support the 'lowest possible dose for the shortest amount of time' approach to treatment. Since we always want to minimize potential side effects, we start low and adjust dosing based off symptom response. We don't use the lowest dose, we use the lowest dose that is *effective at relieving symptoms*. The goal is improved quality of life, and as long as the benefits outweigh the risks for you, you can continue therapy for as long as it's beneficial for you."

Experts and professional organizations agree with the evidence, which increasingly points to continuing MHT past the age of 65 as long as it still benefits the patient, as it may reduce risks of certain cancers and continue to alleviate symptoms. Like all things menopause (and all medications in general), a woman deserves continuous, comprehensive conversations with her healthcare provider at any age. And like all medications, MHT may have risks. Fortunately, many of the providers I spoke with pointed out that its risks tend to decrease after the first year of use. They also said things like: "I want to be buried with my estrogen patch," if that gives you some perspective!

Prioritize Yourself and Your Healthcare

What does this all mean for women, practically? That for you to get the healthcare you deserve, you must have and maintain an open dialogue with your healthcare providers. It means that you must also be in tune with your body and mood. Now, during perimenopause, postmenopause, forever. I can't emphasize enough the need to take care of yourself by paying attention to yourself, and then seeking help from professionals, especially at pivotal moments of transition.

Some general healthcare guidelines* to follow as you enter midlife include:

- See your primary care physician annually (or more frequently if indicated).
    - » Stay up-to-date with immunizations like the flu shot and other vaccines that are recommended for you.

---

* Guidelines are regularly updated by professional organizations like the American Cancer Society. You can also check the US Department of Health & Human Services' Office on Women's Health "Healthy Living by Age" website for tips on what to ask your doctor in each decade, available at https://womenshealth.gov/healthy-living-age.

- » Get your blood pressure checked at your annual primary care visit; if it's elevated, ask for tips on how to reduce it and when to have it rechecked.
- » Ask for cholesterol screenings by age 45 (if you have known risk factors for heart disease, ask for them earlier). In particular, ask about your lipid profile; remember that "bad" cholesterol (LDL) levels tend to increase during menopause and can increase the risk of cardiovascular disease.
- » Screen for prediabetes and diabetes every three years, starting as early as age 35 if you are overweight or have a family history.
- » Request a bone density test by age 65. Request it as early as age 50 if you have an increased risk of osteoporosis due to factors including early menopause, a family history, a bone fracture after age 50, or history of certain medical conditions like rheumatoid arthritis or thyroid imbalances.
- See your OB/GYN annually (or more frequently if indicated).
  - » Screen for cervical cancer every three years via a Pap smear and pelvic exam and every five years via an HPV test.
- Have an eye exam every two to four years or as indicated.
  - » Think about how many people you know in their 40s who now need reading glasses—you may be next!
- Visit the dentist for an exam and cleaning at least once a year.
  - » They should also do an oral cancer screening—and call attention to any tooth and gum issues that, as we've learned, could be due to perimenopause!
- Visit a dermatologist for full-body professional skin exams, ideally every year if you are higher risk due to a family or personal history of skin cancer, or every two to three years if you are low risk.

> » It's also usually recommended to engage in monthly self-checks, since skin cancer is highly curable if found early. If you notice anything new, different, or unusual, like a new growth or a spot that continues to itch or bleed, get seen by a qualified professional.

- At 40, start screening for breast cancer with a yearly mammogram if you are at average risk of breast cancer. If your mom or sister experienced breast cancer, start with a mammogram 10 years before the age at which she was diagnosed. If you have dense breasts, explore additional screening options like ultrasounds and, if needed, a biopsy. Early detection is key.
- At 45, start screening for colorectal cancer if you are at average risk (at 40 if you have a family history, or 10 years before the age of your family member's diagnosis, whichever is earlier).

And remember, you are an individual with specific needs and risks. Talk to your provider about what that means for you when it comes to screenings. And certainly, talk to them if you aren't feeling good.

I know it's hard to get to the doctor or clinic. I know it can be expensive, time-consuming, or just feel too difficult to get away from work or childcare or both to fit in an appointment. I know you have a lot going on.

But, I also know that you *must* take care of yourself now to be healthy later. "When you're older, you don't want to be a burden—on your kids, on the government, whatever it is. You want to be able to take care of yourself for as long as possible," urged Dr Mandelberger. "So, start now—and remember it's never too late to start."

Yeah, yeah, you might be thinking. I admit, I do this sometimes too. It feels like adding to the mental load when I add to my to-do list to pursue healthcare appointments. It's easy for me to give my clients and friends advice about prioritizing themselves (and I mean it) but then it can be hard to take my own advice. As a working parent of young kids—as a millennial who feels preoccupied with family, friends, career, the state of the world, the state of my messy house—I relate to all women of my generation and beyond who may be thinking, *Who has the time to take care of me?*

But the time, my friends, has got to be now.

Chapter 15

MILLENOPAUSE

• • • • • • • • • • • • • • •

I know we just talked about what's next, about what's coming for us in the future, but now I want to hop into the DeLorean and bring us back to the present.

If you are like a few 30-something friends of mine, you may be thinking, *Why do I have to worry about any of this now? I want to deal with it when I get there and I'm not there yet.* And honestly, that's fine! This book is here for when you need it. My goal is not to worry you about what may happen in the future but to prepare you for what is inevitable so that you're not caught off guard like many of my clients and friends have expressed feeling. My goal is to set you up with information and resources so that you can successfully advocate for what you need when the time comes. My goal is for you to feel like you are not alone.

So let's pause and focus on the here and now, an essential tenet of mindfulness sometimes referred to as "nonstriving" (as in, be with yourself here, now, without actively trying to change anything). Mindfulness, we've learned, can be extremely beneficial in navigating all the changes the menopause transition may bring.

To do so, focus on being where you are and doing one thing at a time. This can include focusing on the food you are eating, the ground beneath your feet as you are walking, or the smell of the fresh air around you as you take a moment to breathe. Such an approach can reduce stress and help one appreciate the joy in life. As my friend and meditation teacher Cheryl Brause described, "The present moment is all you have and the only place you ever live. It's so valuable to find contentment just being where you are!"

Brause and Stephanie Falk cofounded Pause to be Present, a mindfulness studio that in 2024 held, in collaboration with menopause-focused registered dietitian nutritionist Daria Ventura, a menopause education series featuring various experts. Their goal was to create a space where women could learn, share, and connect about this typically taboo topic. They recognized the value of mindfulness and the void in information sought by women in any phase of the menopause transition. "Simply learning to use your breath to relax your nervous system can be very helpful for women," explained Falk. "Training your brain not to worry or perseverate about all the symptoms or issues you are experiencing or that you may experience down the road is incredibly useful for women, whether they are premenopausal, perimenopausal, or postmenopausal."

Brause added: "Stress reduction is a very important tool to address so many of the symptoms of menopause, because stress often exacerbates the symptoms. Understanding how we can regulate our nervous systems and reduce our levels of cortisol (the body's main stress hormone) is a huge benefit of mindfulness and meditation." She teaches meditation practices that help us slow down, relax, and focus our minds in healthy ways.

Mindfulness is accessible to people of all backgrounds and is promoted by menopause healthcare providers of all fields. For example, Mindfulness-Based Stress Reduction (MBSR) is a therapeutic tool that has been proved to improve the level of mindfulness and relieve anxiety symptoms in menopausal women with severe symptoms like hot flashes or insomnia.[281] Dr. Hausvater noted that mindfulness, cognitive behavioral therapy, deep breathing, and meditation can benefit hearth health: "These tools can help improve sleep, and poor sleep is a very important risk factor associated with higher blood pressure, obesity, and other issues linked to heart disease." Dr. Bhopal agreed: "Relaxation and coping skills, including mindfulness, breathwork, and muscle relaxation, can help improve breathing. And how you breathe has such a big impact on how you feel and sleep."

Gentle, mindful yoga can be a helpful practice to implement to improve sleep. Dr. Ashley Austin, the sports physician, also appreciates the benefits of yoga for the health at midlife: "I really like yoga and Pilates as mindful exercises that help women." Research confirms that mind-body exercises like yoga and Pilates can positively influence bone mineral density, sleep quality, and mental health among perimenopausal and postmenopausal women.[282]

"Yoga fundamentally changed my life," shared yoga therapist Fiona Jalinoos. In addition to pelvic floor therapy and hormone therapy, she has personally found that Hatha yoga, a slow-paced technique that focuses on energy, has been integral to her feeling balanced throughout perimenopause. She now helps other women practice yoga, mindfulness, and acceptance. "Learn what you can control, and let go of what you can't," Jalinoos encouraged. "Yoga helps us work with ourselves, not against ourselves. It helps us send our energy in the right direction. Mindful yoga helps with distress tolerance."

Indeed, mindfulness is also a tool that therapists like me and other wellness practitioners like to use to ease anxiety over what might happen in the future. It helps us focus on the here and now and reminds us that we can control only what we can control. As Falk described, "Simply asking yourself, 'What is happening to my body today and what can I do to try and feel better?' can help ease the stories in our heads. Worrying about the future or about what happened in the past can cause many women lots of extra stress and anxiety, and focusing on the present helps alleviate that."

We can also feel better by treating ourselves (and our peers) with kindness and pride. "Women at midlife who embrace the value of their life experiences have so much less tolerance for bullshit—in a good way!" observed Randi Zinn, founder of The Group Experience, a program through which she facilitates supportive groups for women, including "Midlife Magic" groups for women ages 40 to 65. "Your life at this time may not be exactly what you had expected, but if you accept it as reality, you can let go a bit and recognize that 'unexpected' or 'challenging' doesn't necessarily mean 'bad.' You can not only get through hard times but also thrive."

HOW CAN MILLENNIALS PREPARE?

Be Mindful

Start by implementing a mindfulness practice—today! Be intentional when you're walking, moving, eating, or engaging in everyday tasks. Try a five-minute meditation (please believe me, you can squeeze in five minutes as a start).

I understand if you are reluctant. It might sound a little woo-woo, or you might be telling yourself that you have no time for this kind of "unproductive" activity. I totally get it. I felt the same for most of my life, despite always appreciating mystical vibes. But it wasn't just the literature I reviewed or the expert guidance I received that convinced me to embrace mindfulness over the last several years—it was also the appreciation I began to feel for the here and now, the changes I've seen in my clients' mental health and my own, the joy I leaned into when my kids begged for nighttime back tickles while my to-do list remained long. It's a real gift to yourself to be able to mute the swirling hum of the mental load and just be present. I promise.

So what can we do now, in this present moment? Pause. Breathe. Check in with your body. Check in with your mental health. Check in with how you feel, physically, mentally, and emotionally.

Consider any changes and if those changes are impacting you. "Women tend to tell themselves, 'Oh this is just life, it's busy and stressful, and of course I feel kind of crappy,'" Dr. Hertel said she observes in her millennial patients who complain, *I don't feel like myself*. "But I always ask patients to consider—did you feel this way when you were super stressed in school? At work? Yes, life can be stressful but there may be something else going on that is making you react differently, and that may be perimenopause."

She, like all of the experts I got to know through my research, encourages women to get support throughout their menopause journeys. "Every single one of us can benefit from lifestyle optimization now," encouraged Dr. Mandelberger. "And, if desired, women should seek treatment for issues that are bothersome or interfering with quality of life. As a culture we tend to resist aging, but I think we are better off embracing inevitable changes than denying them."

And for now, menopause is very much inevitable and not preventable. Research is currently being conducted at Columbia University on whether ovarian function can be slowed, thereby delaying menopause and improving longevity.[283] When I spoke with fertility specialists like Drs. Taraneh Nazem and Arielle Bayer, they expressed curiosity and interest in such research because of potential health benefits—but reminded me that women are not meant to be pregnant in older ages like their 70s and 80s because it's not safe. And of course, our value as women extends beyond just baby-making! Agreed Anne Fulenwider of Alloy: "Some women welcome menopause, welcome the end of their period and childbearing years. Women may just want to live healthfully in this new phase of life. And they deserve to be able to with safe, affordable options."

Be Kind to Yourself

Mindfulness and other cognitive behavioral therapy tools like acceptance and commitment therapy (ACT) can help women accept their symptoms without judgment and move through them. A positive outlook can be immensely helpful during the menopause transition.[284] "You're better off being nice to yourself about what your new norm is," advised Mirchandani. Research confirms that a positive or at least neutral attitude is beneficial when approaching menopause, as negative views of the transition have been linked to experiencing more symptoms.[285] So while venting or sitting with your negative feelings can be temporarily helpful (I love a good release through crying!), accepting your present life status through mindfulness may be worth pursuing as an overall strategy as you approach this phase.

In fact, mindfulness is a great tool to use during any transitional period. "It helps us learn to accept inevitable changes and acknowledge they are a normal part of aging. With openness, we can navigate the changes with greater acceptance. Instead of resisting, we can embrace this time of life and take control of our health," Brause suggested. Mindfulness can also help us truly accept the fact that aging—despite the struggles that might come with it—is a privilege. A lot of people, due to any number of misfortunes, don't have the opportunity to grow old. If you can reframe your thoughts to welcome each new year or new life period, menopause and other transitions won't be so daunting.

Along with changes, menopause can bring opportunities for women. And I think we all have an opportunity here and now to reframe what being an older woman actually looks like. Sarah Shealy, the nurse midwife and menopause practitioner, often draws upon other cultures, like in China where she lived for a few years, that revere and respect older women. The US is not quite there, but maybe it can be soon.

"Our society has bought into the idea of an aging woman as one who is at the end of being attractive or sexual or valuable," noted Jannine Versi of Elektra. "So we get the message that life is over at menopause, that it is just painful and downhill from here." I hope after reading most of this book you now know and wholeheartedly believe that's just not true. Think of how many women you know in their 50s and beyond who are thriving. You can be one of them! Damn the man who tries to tell us otherwise. Jo Piazza, the author and journalist, agreed: "For too long women have been told that each decade represents a shriveling away of our place in the world, that we will get smaller and sadder and less impactful. This is a lie perpetuated mostly by men, probably because they have long been afraid of the power and vitality of women as we age."

Let's lean in to our power, ladies. Perhaps we can think of this time as a gift. To draw upon a quotation too many of us used in our high school yearbooks, it's called "the present" for a reason, isn't it?

Dr. Kathy Casey, the acupuncture and Eastern medicine provider, does think of menopause that way, believing that menopause is an opportunity to embrace the change the present moment offers. "Being open to change, recognizing there is a time and a season for all things—and learning how to be with what is—reflects the Taoist philosophy. We can emphasize living in accord with nature and the natural way of things. We can choose, as women, to return to our inner knowing, our own guiding light—to awaken and reconnect with our True Self. This is the gift of the menopausal transition."

As we go through this natural life transition, we can and should continue to rely on each other for resources. There are few things more powerful than women in community together. Courtney Mamuscia, a marketing expert based in Denver, was inspired to build an online community specifically to ensure that women dealing with menopause felt like they had support. She launched a podcast, *Hot Flash Health*, with Dawn Fable in 2024. "Menopause doesn't have to be a lonely, confusing, or frustrating journey," insists their website, geared toward a midlife woman who identifies as a "queenager" (love it!). Mamuscia explained: "Our goal is to create a platform where women feel safe to embrace their full selves. Menopause should not be a secret. It's something we all go through and can't get away from. So, let's own it and accept it. We want to hype women up for this next phase of life!"

Kara Cruz, the therapist, noted that in her groups, "Women share books, screening tools, webinars, and experiences. They hold each other accountable in asserting themselves and teach each other what questions to ask at their healthcare appointments." Such connection is incredibly meaningful and can be found not only in professional support groups but also in conversations with peers and older women, the growing media resources in this space, and professional and social networks. Strike up a chat with another woman in the doctor's office waiting room or in the section of the store where you got this book. Remember, you are not alone!

I understand if you're feeling fear around menopause in general, though I don't intend to be way harsh or fill you with an overwhelming sense of ickiness. Instead, I encourage you to be inquisitive and even maybe enthusiastic. Research reflects that women who have made it through the transition view menopause more positively than those currently in the thick of it,[286] as is the case with many intimidating events for which we tend to have anticipatory anxiety. "Menopause is nothing to be afraid of," Shealy, Duke, and so many of the women's health experts I interviewed insisted.

Taking a lighthearted approach can be helpful, too. Menopause can be messy but doesn't need to be so defining or consuming. "I think you have to laugh about it sometimes," my family friend Karen reflected. "It's life, it happens! You may have bad days, but there is so much you can do to help yourself feel better. Keep trying different things until you do!" And keep finding small reasons to smile, even on hard days. So many women I spoke with, including those just a few years older than I who were born in the 1970s, shared that the menopause transition can genuinely bring about a lot of joy.

Menopause, like Mama Beasts' Hemphill described, can be a time to think of "your body calling you back in. This is truly an opportunity to take care of your health and prioritize yourself." I love thinking about the menopause transition as a time of opportunity. It's an opportunity to approach your life with self-assuredness and strength. It's an opportunity to lift up yourself and other women. It's an opportunity for empowerment!

My friend Kyle Koeppel Mann, for whom menopause was induced at age 34, does view menopause positively. "I feel empowered," she explained, "in that I don't have to worry about an undetectable cancer the same way I did before my surgery. The choices I made about my healthcare, about when and how to have my family, and about how to take care of my body and health were my own. I feel grateful that I went through menopause."

My paternal grandmother, Ilene, likewise told me that she very much experienced a feeling of empowerment back when she went through menopause, which she, too, chose to have surgically induced. Shortly before her 94th birthday, we had a conversation that went like this:

"Grandma, I'm writing a book! I've been so excited to tell you."

"Oh, darling, I'm so happy for you. If I could jump up and down, I would."

"It's about menopause and my generation."

"Well, that's very important. I got my ovaries and uterus removed at 35 because I didn't want to deal with that shit. I had horrible cramps every month and I was so relieved to no longer get my period. I insisted that the doctor do the procedure because I was so done with all that, so ready for menopause."

"Thank you for telling me."

"You go write that book. I don't believe that women should suffer for one second. If they have any kind of pain, or need any kind of help, they should get support. Women deserve support. You go tell them."

I hope that I have told you, through this book. I hope I've made her proud.

Conclusion

HOW CAN MILLENNIALS PREPARE FOR MENOPAUSE?

In truth, there is no one way to prepare for menopause. I've learned and shared with you lots of information, resources, and things to think about, hoping they are helpful as you navigate what's next. There is truly no one-size-fits-all approach to this next phase. And I am not here to preach about how to be a pillar of health. TBH, I still love drinking Diet Coke and the look of a suntan.

But I am here to remind you—and myself—that women deserve opportunities to take care of themselves and to change a world that won't support them in doing so.

You may still be skeptical. *Me? Menopause? I'm so far away from that and don't need to think about it yet.* But menopause experts are increasingly calling for healthcare providers to have more conversations with women beginning at age 35, to help them anticipate the menopause transition and establish an ongoing dialogue about symptoms and treatment preferences. As of 2025, I'm 40, and no provider has ever proactively raised the subject of perimenopause with me. To the contrary, when I've broached the issue, I've been met with dismissive "You're too young to worry about that" remarks. I'm not worried (or crazy or being dramatic, like women are too often portrayed to be)—I'm just curious. And I'll keep asking questions, for myself, for my clients, for my peers, and for you.

Somewhat on the flip side, you may be skeptical about whether "perimenopause" is too readily offered as the answer to all of your problems and why discussions on the menopause transition suddenly seem to be everywhere. *Are my issues really menopause-related, or is this diagnosis a distracting trend?* I literally laughed upon learning that common perimenopause symptoms include fatigue, worsening memory, and metabolism changes—things nearly every millennial woman I know complains about. It's ironic, don't ya think? Several friends have recently said to me: "Maybe it's because we've been talking about your book, but my algorithm keeps feeding me content about perimenopause." I'm with you; I'm now getting ads on LinkedIn from AARP claiming, "Menopause is stealing your hottest talent" (cute). A woman born in 1979 told me upon hearing about my research: "Perimenopause feels like avocado felt a few years ago—suddenly it's everywhere, but really, it was in front of us all along." I've seen the memes and can make my own: If you ever tried the Snooki hair poof look, if your first crush was on Dylan or Brandon, if you collected Absolut ads in binders or Lisa Frank puffy stickers in scrapbooks… You might be in perimenopause.

"Might be" is the key phrase here. Hormone shifts are not responsible for everything. If your sleep has been interrupted lately, it might be due to perimenopausal night sweats—or to a sleep disorder. If you're feeling irritable more often than not, it might be due to perimenopausal mood swings—or to being fed up with discrimination against women. If you're experiencing cloudy memories or distractedness, it might be due to perimenopausal brain fog—or to overwhelm from all the invisible, undervalued cognitive labor you're doing.

Symptoms may be due to aging in general, or to the inequitable treatment women endure, or to menopause specifically, or to some combination of these experiences.

Whatever it is you're going through, you deserve support and information.

As a psychotherapist, labels can be helpful, but I prioritize treating the symptoms to help my clients feel better. As an advocate, I strive to improve access to healthcare and achieve gender equity in the home, in the workplace, and beyond. As a mom, I aspire to instill in my children the values of compassion and generosity. As a woman, I hope that I can lean on other women for support and they can likewise depend on me, as I firmly believe we are stronger together.

For millennials approaching midlife, whether already actively managing the menopause transition or not, here are my simplified suggested strategies for preparing for life's next period.

- **INVESTIGATE**

  You are the expert on your own body and mental health. If you begin to feel unlike yourself, take note. Track your periods, your moods, your physical symptoms, and anything else that feels off or new. Keeping a record helps us see patterns, triggers, and signs more clearly.

- **COMMUNICATE**

  And then talk about it. Admit what's going on to yourself, tell your friends or other trusted confidants, and inform your healthcare providers. If you feel uncomfortable, find a provider who makes you feel safe and/or get support from loved ones or professionals to articulate your needs. We must speak up and speak out if we want to be heard.

- **EDUCATE**

  So many women are self-taught about menopause and other issues deemed "women's health" because too little attention to these issues is paid by mainstream media and medicine. Keep learning, keep inquiring, keep sharing. Educate yourself on family history and genetics and on the latest research and offerings. If you end up like me, with an opportunity to teach your own doctors about innovative treatment options, embrace it. We're all learning together.

- **PARTICIPATE**

    Your relationship with your provider should be a partnership. Respecting self-determination is part of a social worker's code of ethics, and I believe that all healthcare providers must respect a woman's autonomy to make her own choices. There are so many nuances to menopause, we now know. You must be able to trust your provider, to feel like they truly listen to and see you. With all of the healthcare options out there (and more on their way), you must be able to engage in shared decision-making about what to try and when, how to wean off or resume or adjust medication if desired, and what your goals are.

- **EVALUATE**

    What's right for one woman or even one moment may not be right for the next when it comes to treatment for symptom relief or lifestyle modifications. I could add "meditate, medicate, and/or fornicate" here because they are all valid options, as alternatives or complements to each other. We've learned that hormone therapy is considered the gold standard approach to menopause symptoms and is generally safe and effective, but not everyone needs or wants to take it, even if they can. A friend born in 1986 noticed experiencing wild mood swings around ovulation but didn't like how birth control made her feel; instead of meds, she got a handle on her symptoms by implementing behavioral strategies like seeking alone time and drinking lots of water before getting her period. Good for her! You should do what feels right for you, for right now. Continue to check in with yourself and modify as needed.

- **ADVOCATE**

    If you are told that feeling chronically wiped out is just a part of life now, push back. If you are told that you can't be in perimenopause because your periods are still regular, or because you're too young, or because your hormone levels appear normal in your blood work, push back. If you are told that middle-aged women are unattractive characters in media, that companies for women's health are not worth investing in, or that workplaces should not care about menopause, push back. We must raise the next generation to care more about women. We must convince our own generation that women deserve better. Share the information you've learned with males in your life. Vote for lawmakers who will actually represent your interests. Advocate for yourself by prioritizing quality of life and advocate for all women by insisting on individualized, quality care. As my queen Jenny sang in 1999, let's get loud.

- **VALIDATE**

    Just because common symptoms or experiences may be common does not mean you have to suffer through them. You should get the care you deserve (for menopause or otherwise). Additionally, you should support other women, even if their experience is vastly different from your own. Much of this book discusses treatment options for women of average general health and assumes access to certain resources. More research is being done—and needed—on the menopause transition and women who live in rural areas, women who identify as LGBTQ+, women with a disability, and more. There is still so much more to learn. Far too many women are underserved by our healthcare and other systems, including those who may have experienced illness, speak another language, or are struggling to break a cycle of generational poverty. All deserve recognition and support.

- **ELEVATE**

  One of the best parts of writing this book has been joining a community of like-minded women who want to help women feel empowered as they experience the menopause transition. The dozens of experts I've gotten to know—whether they work in healthcare, law, or finance, or have just chosen to share their experiences to assist others—have been genuinely kind and collaborative. We are truly all in this together. It is sincerely my honor to be able to uplift the work and passions of other women. As millennial Serena Williams has said: "The success of every woman should be the inspiration to another. We should raise each other up."

- **APPRECIATE**

  Menopause is, by definition, a life transition. It's natural to feel ambivalent about the changes you are experiencing, the shifts in your identity. But how beautiful is it to have had a time in your life that you are sad is ending? How wonderful might it feel to accept the opportunity for something new rather than resist it? You've heard from some of my many friends who have survived cancer or live with genetic mutations that put their health at risk; they and others with autoimmune conditions or who have endured trauma constantly remind me to appreciate the moment, appreciate my health. I encourage us all to adopt that mindset when it comes to menopause.

- **CELEBRATE**

    Aging can be… a lot, I acknowledge that. But we'll never be as young as we are now. And deep down, we'll always be girls who just wanna have fun! Maybe every day can be as special as Rex Manning Day if we approach it that way and release our inhibitions. For a recent not-so-big birthday, for example, I invited 80 of my closest girlfriends to wear whatever they felt most fabulous in, eat various forms of french fries, and dance to early aughts pop music; it felt light and fun and much needed after a year marked by tragedy in the world and in our town. It reminded me that we can always find something in life to celebrate.

And we can find something about menopause to celebrate, too. Many, many women have described the postmenopause period as one in which they feel wise, proud, resilient, vibrant, comfortable with themselves, more intentional, less of a people pleaser, powerful, and positive. Menopause does not need to be a negative experience, and hopefully isn't one, if you feel prepared for it and open to it.

One of my favorite mindfulness exercises is a gratitude practice, in which one focuses on the good things in one's life, big or small. I am grateful that we are learning and talking more about menopause and women's health. I am grateful that women are coming together to demand better and are being kind to each other. I am grateful to you for being here. Let's enjoy ourselves!

Menopause is the end of a period in life.

And, it's the beginning of another.

RESOURCES AND ADDITIONAL READING

Keep learning! Below are some of my favorite resources and other relevant reading materials.

(This is not an exhaustive list; check out each chapter's cited resources for even more, and please feel free to get in touch with additional suggestions.)

RESOURCES

- The International Society for the Study of Women's Sexual Health (ISSWSH)
  https://www.isswsh.org

- The Menopause Society
  https://menopause.org

  » The Menopause Society's searchable directory of trained menopause practitioners is available at https://portal.menopause.org/NAMS/NAMS/Directory/Menopause-Practitioner.aspx

- The Women's Mental Health Consortium (WMHC)
  https://wmhcny.org

ADDITIONAL READING

- Bluming, Avrum, and Carol Tavris. *Estrogen Matters: Why Taking Hormones in Menopause Can Improve Women's Well-Being and Lengthen Their Lives—Without Raising the Risk of Breast Cancer.* Little, Brown Spark, 2024.

- Kay, Katty, and Claire Shipman. *The Confidence Code: The Science and Art of Self-Assurance—What Women Should Know.* Harper Business, 2018.

- Tang, Karen. *It's Not Hysteria: Everything You Need to Know About Your Reproductive Health.* Flatiron Books, 2024.

- Waldman, Emily Gold, Bridget J. Crawford, and Naomi R. Cahn. *Hot Flash: How the Law Ignores Menopause and What We Can Do About It*. Stanford University Press, 2024.

ENDNOTES

Introduction

1 Michael Dimock, "Defining Generations: Where Millennials End and Generation Z Begins," Pew Research Center, January 17, 2019, https://www.pewresearch.org/short-reads/2019/01/17/where-millennials-end-and-generation-z-begins.

2 "Premature Menopause," The Menopause Society, accessed December 12, 2024, https://menopause.org/patient-education/menopause-topics/premature-menopause.

3 K. Hill, "The Demography of Menopause," *Maturitas* 23, no. 2 (1996): 113, DOI: 10.1016/0378-5122(95)00968-x.

4 "Life Expectancy," Centers for Disease Control, last updated October 25, 2024, https://www.cdc.gov/nchs/fastats/life-expectancy.htm.

Chapter 1

5 Melinda Wenner Moyer, "'Turning Red' Is a Good Conversation Starter—and Not Just for Girls," *The New York Times*, March 16, 2022,

https://www.nytimes.com/2022/03/16/well/family/turning-red-periods-discussion.html.

6   "State of the Period 2023," PERIOD.org, accessed October 15, 2024, https://period.org/uploads/2023-State-of-the-Period-Study.pdf.

Chapter 2

7   See: Lauren A. Tetenbaum, "Are You There, Menopause? It's Me, a Millennial Mom," MamaBeasts.com, March 7, 2024, https://www.mamabeasts.com/articles/are-you-there-menopause-its-me-a-millennial-mom.

8   C. Munn et al., "Menopause Knowledge and Education in Women under 40: Results from an Online Survey," *Women's Health* (London) 18 (2022), DOI: 10.1177/17455057221139660.

9   Learn more: Jane L. Yang et al., "Estrogen Deficiency in the Menopause and the Role of Hormone Therapy: Integrating the Findings of Basic Science Research with Clinical Trials," *Menopause* 31, no. 10 (2024): 926–39, DOI: 10.1097/GME.0000000000002407.

10   See, e.g.: Maria Godoy, "Girls Are Getting Their First Periods Earlier. Here's What Parents Should Know," *NPR*, May 31, 2024, https://www.npr.org/sections/shots-health-news/2024/05/31/nx-s1-4985074/girls-are-getting-their-first-periods-earlier-heres-what-parents-should-know.

11   Carolyn J. Crandall et al., *Menopause Practice: A Clinician's Guide*, 6th Edition (The North American Menopause Society, 2023).

12   "The State of Perimenopause in 2024," Oova, accessed March 2024, https://view.ceros.com/oova/state-of-perimenopause-report-landing-page/p/1.

13   See, e.g.: Cynthia A. Stuenkel, "What Is Menopause?" *Menopause* 31, no. 9 (2024): 837–8, DOI: 10.1097/GME.0000000000002416.

14   Learn more: Fiona C. Baker et al., "Sleep Problems During the Menopausal Transition: Prevalence, Impact, and Management Challenges," *Nature and Science of Sleep* 10 (2018): 73–95, DOI: 10.2147/NSS.S125807.

15   See, e.g.: Christina A. Metcalf et al., "Cognitive Problems in Perimenopause: A Review of Recent Evidence," *Current Psychiatry Reports* 25, no. 10 (2023): 501, DOI: 10.1007/s11920-023-01447-3.

16   "Premature Menopause," The Menopause Society.

17   See, e.g.: Kira von Eichel, "Extreme Stress Can Trigger Early Menopause," *Oprah Daily*, August 4, 2023, https://www.oprahdaily.com/life/health/a44664881/early-menopause-period-end-of-story.

18   Ellen B. Gold et al., "Longitudinal Analysis of the Association between Vasomotor Symptoms and Race/Ethnicity across the Menopausal Transition: Study of Women's Health Across the Nation," *American Journal of Public Health* 96, no. 7 (2006): 1226–35, DOI: 10.2105/AJPH.2005.066936.

19   Alexis N. Reeves et al., "Does Everyday Discrimination Account for the Increased Risk of Vasomotor Symptoms in Black Women? The Study of Women's Health Across The Nation (SWAN)," *Menopause* 31, no. 6 (2024): 484–93, DOI: 10.1097/GME.0000000000002357.

20   Alison Kochersberger et al., "The Association of Race, Ethnicity, and Socioeconomic Status on the Severity of Menopause Symptoms: A Study of 68,864 Women," *Menopause* 31, no. 6 (2024): 476–83, DOI: 10.1097/GME.0000000000002349.

21   Juanita J. Chinn et al., "Health Equity Among Black Women in the United States," *Journal of Women's Health* 30, no. 2 (2021): 212, DOI: 10.1089/jwh.2020.8868.

22   See, e.g.: Alisah Haridasani Gupta, "How Menopause Affects Women of Color," *The New York Times*, last updated September 4, 2023, https://www.nytimes.com/2023/08/23/well/live/menopause-symptoms-women-of-color.html.

23   See, e.g.: Meryl Sebastian and Anagha Pathak, "Menopause, the Other Menstrual Taboo for Indian Women," *BBC News*, November 13, 2024, https://bbc.com/news/articles/ce8dzjyp4p8o?mc_cid=9256962ac7&mc_eid=b599d04e73.

Chapter 3

24   Michael J. Glantz et al., "Gender Disparity in the Rate of Partner Abandonment in Patients with Serious Medical Illness," *Cancer* 115, no. 22 (2009): 5237–42, DOI: 10.1002/cncr.24577.

25   Jacques E. Rossouw, "Risks and Benefits of Estrogen plus Progestin in Healthy Postmenopausal Women: Principal Results from the Women's Health Initiative Randomized Controlled Trial," *The Journal of the American Medical Association* 288, no. 3 (2002): 321–33, DOI: 10.1001/jama.288.3.32.

26 See also: S. Richards, "Hormone Therapy Was Villainized for Decades. Now, It's Back, But Who Really Should Be On It?" *Women's Health*, October 30, 2024, https://www.womenshealthmag.com/health/a62734967/hormone-therapy-who-should-take-it.

27 Nick Panay et al., "Menopause and MHT in 2024: Addressing the Key Controversies—an International Menopause Society White Paper," *Climacteric* 27, no. 5 (2024): 441–57, DOI: 10.1080/13697137.2024.2394950.

28 "Hormone Therapy Usage Rates Still Low Despite Proven Benefits," The Menopause Society, September 10, 2024, https://menopause.org/wp-content/uploads/press-release/HT-Use-Stagnant.pdf.

29 See, e.g.: Angelo Cagnacci and Martina Venier, "The Controversial History of Hormone Replacement Therapy," *Medicina* 55, no. 9 (2019): 602, DOI: 10.3390/medicina55090602.

30 Stephanie Sy and Courtney Norris, "Hormone Replacement Safe and Effective Menopause Treatment, Study Finds," *PBS*, May 6, 2024, https://www.pbs.org/newshour/show/hormone-replacement-safe-and-effective-menopause-treatment-study-finds. See also: S. Dominus, "Women Have Been Misled about Menopause," *The New York Times*, last updated June 15, 2023, https://www.nytimes.com/2023/02/01/magazine/menopause-hot-flashes-hormone-therapy.html.

31 Jennifer Wolff, "What Doctors Don't Know About Menopause," *AARP The Magazine*, September 2018, www.hopkinsmedicine.org/-/media/womens-wellness-program/what_doctors_dont_know_about_menopause-aarp.

32 Juliana M. Kling et al., "Menopause Management Knowledge in Postgraduate Family Medicine, Internal Medicine, and Obstetrics and Gynecology Residents: A Cross-Sectional Survey," *Mayo Clinic Proceedings* 94, no. 2 (2019): 242, DOI: 10.1016/j.mayocp.2018.08.033.

33 Jennifer T. Allen et al., "Needs Assessment of Menopause Education in United States Obstetrics and Gynecology Residency Training Programs," *Menopause* 30, no. 10 (2023): 1002–05, DOI: 10.1097/GME.0000000000002234.

34 "Hormone Therapy Usage Rates Still Low Despite Proven Benefits," The Menopause Society.

35   Angela Garbes, "Perimenopause Has Brought Chaos to My Life—but Also Peace," *The Guardian*, March 27, 2024, https://www.theguardian.com/wellness/2024/mar/27/perimenopause-life-changes.

36   See, e.g.: Cassandra Roeca et al., "The Postmenopausal Women," in *Endotext* (Endotext, 2018), https://www.ncbi.nlm.nih.gov/books/NBK279131/; Cagnacci and Venier, "The Controversial History of Hormone Replacement Therapy"; Stephanie S. Faubion et al., "The 2022 Hormone Therapy Position Statement of the North American Menopause Society," *Menopause* 29, no. 7 (2022): 767–94, DOI: 10.1097/GME.0000000000002028

37   JoAnn E. Manson et al., "Menopausal Hormone Therapy and Health Outcomes During the Intervention and Extended Poststopping Phases of the Women's Health Initiative Randomized Trials," *The Journal of the American Medical Association* 310, no. 13 (2013): 1353–68, DOI:10.1001/jama.2013.278040.

38   Nancy Shute, "The Last Word on Hormone Therapy from the Women's Health Initiative," *NPR*, October 4, 2013, https://www.npr.org/sections/health-shots/2013/10/04/229171477/the-last-word-on-hormone-therapy-from-the-womens-health-initiative.

39   Wolff, "What Doctors Don't Know About Menopause."

40   "The Women's Health Initiative (WHI) Reports Key Findings and Clinical Messages from Long-Term Follow-Up," Brigham and Women's Hospital, May 1, 2024, https://www.brighamandwomens.org/about-bwh/newsroom/press-releases-detail?id=4701, citing JoAnn E. Manson et al., "The Women's Health Initiative Randomized Trials and Clinical Practice," *The Journal of the American Medical Association* 331, no. 20 (2024): 1748–60, DOI:10.1001/jama.2024.6542.

41   See, e.g.: "Delayed Diagnosis and Treatment of Menopause Is Wasting NHS Appointments and Resources," balance-menopause.com, June 30, 2021, https://www.balance-menopause.com/news/delayed-diagnosis-and-treatment-of-menopause-is-wasting-nhs-appointments-and-resources; Jessie Van Amburg, "Nearly 1 in 3 Women Have Had Their Menopause Symptoms Misdiagnosed," OurKindra.com, accessed September 28, 2024, https://ourkindra.com/blogs/journal/menopause-medical-misdiagnosis.

42   See also: Mary Claire Haver, "Out of Touch on Menopause: Experts Respond to The Lancet's 'Over-Medicalization' Claims." *Ms. Magazine*,

April 15, 2024, https://msmagazine.com/2024/04/15/menopause-treatment-the-lancet.

Chapter 4

43 See also: Lauren Streicher, "Invisible Women Syndrome," *Dr. Streicher's Inside Information: THE Menopause Podcast*, November 13, 2024, https://www.iheart.com/podcast/270-dr-streichers-inside-infor-94545667/episode/s3-ep154-invisible-woman-syndrome-238150962.

44 "Attention Marketers: US Women Are Eager to Hear from You," Nielsen, November 2019, https://www.nielsen.com/insights/2019/attention-marketers-u-s-women-are-eager-to-hear-from-you.

45 See, e.g.: Victoria Rideout and S. Craig Watkins, "Millennials, Social Media, and Politics," The University of Texas at Austin, Institute for Media, 2019, https://moody.utexas.edu/sites/default/files/Millennials-Social-Media-Politics.pdf; "How Gen Z and Millennials Use Social Media Differently," MSSMedia.com, last updated March 2024, https://info.mssmedia.com/blog/how-gen-z-and-millennials-use-social-media-differently; Jacqueline Zote, "Social Media Demographics to Inform Your 2024 Strategy," SproutSocial.com, February 14, 2024, https://sproutsocial.com/insights/new-social-media-demographics.

46 See, e.g.: Talker Research, "Study Reveals Lack of Menopause Education Among American Women," *Talker*, October 14, 2024, https://talker.news/2024/10/14/study-reveals-lack-of-menopause-education-among-american-women.

Chapter 5

47 Gretchen Livingston, "They're Waiting Longer, but US Women Today More Likely to Have Children Than a Decade Ago," Pew Research Center, January 18, 2018, https://www.pewresearch.org/social-trends/2018/01/18/theyre-waiting-longer-but-u-s-women-today-more-likely-to-have-children-than-a-decade-ago.

48 See, e.g.: Reyhan Harmanci, "The Truth about Pregnancy over 40," *The New York Times*, last updated March 29, 2022, https://www.nytimes.com/2020/04/15/parenting/pregnancy/baby-after-40.html; Stephanie S. Faubion, "What You Need to Know about Pregnancy after Age 40," *Mayo Clinic*, December 18, 2023, https://mcpress.mayoclinic.org/pregnancy/what-you-need-to-know-about-pregnancy-after-age-40.

49   Rachel E. Gross, "Why So Many Accidental Pregnancies Happen in Your 40s," *The Atlantic*, last updated November 20, 2023, https://www.theatlantic.com/health/archive/2023/11/perimenopause-vs-menopause-age-pregnancy/675998, citing Lauren M. Rossen et al., "Updated Methodology to Estimate Overall and Unintended Pregnancy Rates in the United States," *Vital Health Statistics* 2, no. 201 (2023), DOI: 10.15620/cdc:124395.

50   Jamie Ducharme, "Why So Many Women Are Waiting Longer to Have Kids," *Time*, last updated April 10, 2024, https://time.com/6965267/women-having-kids-later.

Chapter 6

51   Learn more: Barbara Levy and James A. Simon, "A Contemporary View of Menopausal Hormone Therapy," *Obstetrics & Gynecology* 144, no. 1 (2024): 12, DOI: 10.1097/aog.0000000000005553; Dominus, "Women Have Been Misled about Menopause"; Nick Panay et al., "Menopause and MHT in 2024: Addressing the Key Controversies—an International Menopause Society White Paper," *Climacteric* 27, no. 5 (2024): 441–57, DOI: 10.1080/13697137.2024.2394950.

52   Claudio N. Soares, "Depression and Menopause," *Medical Clinics of North America* 103, no. 4 (2019): 651–67, DOI: 10.1016/j.mcna.2019.03.001.

53   Nanette Santoro, "Menopause Step-by-Step: Basics of the Menopause Transition," *Menopause* 31, no. 10 (2024): 921, DOI: 10.1097/GME.0000000000002423.

54   Faubion et al., "The 2022 Hormone Therapy Position Statement."

55   See, e.g.: Let's Talk Menopause, "Menoposium 2024 Panel 2: The Facts about Hormone Therapy with Sharon Malone and Mary Claire Haver," YouTube, June 18, 2024, https://www.youtube.com/watch?v=t2i0BgtrZJ4.

56   American College of Obstetricians and Gynecologists' Committee on Clinical Consensus-Gynecology in collaboration with Amy J. Park and Belinda Yauger (endorsed by The American Society for Reproductive Medicine), "Compounded Bioidentical Menopausal Hormone Therapy," *Obstetrics & Gynecology* 142, no. 5 (2023): 1266, https://www.acog.org/clinical/clinical-guidance/clinical-consensus/articles/2023/11/compounded-bioidentical-menopausal-hormone-therapy.

57   Allison Aubrey, "Hormones for Menopause Are Safe, Study Finds. Here's What Changed," *NPR*, May 1, 2024, https://www.npr.org/sections/health-shots/2024/05/01/1248525256/hormones-menopause-hormone-therapy-hot-flashes.

58   Meredith K. Wise et al., "Public Awareness and Provider Counseling Regarding Postmenopausal Bleeding as a Symptom of Endometrial Cancer," *Menopause* 31, no. 10 (2024): 905–10, DOI: 10.1097/gme.0000000000002411

59   Chris R. Cardwell et al., "Hormone Replacement Therapy and Cancer Mortality in Women with 17 Site-Specific Cancers: A Cohort Study Using Linked Medical Records," *British Journal of Cancer* 131, no. 4 (2024): 737, DOI: 10.1038/s41416-024-02767-8.

60   See, e.g.: Leslie Cho et al., "Rethinking Menopausal Hormone Therapy: For Whom, What, When and How Long?" *Circulation* 147, no. 7 (2023): 597, DOI: 10.1161/CIRCULATIONAHA.122.061559; Faubion et al., "The 2022 Hormone Therapy Position Statement."

61   Faubion et al., "The 2022 Hormone Therapy Position Statement."

62   "The 2023 Nonhormone Therapy Position Statement of the North American Menopause Society," *Menopause* 30, no. 6 (2023): 573–90, DOI: 10.1097/gme.0000000000002200; Alisa Johnson et al., "Complementary and Alternative Medicine for Menopause," *Journal of Evidence-Based Integrative Medicine* 24 (2019), DOI: 10.1177/2515690X19829380.

63   See, e.g.: Myra S. Hunter, "Cognitive Behavioral Therapy for Menopausal Symptoms," *Climacteric* 24, no. 1 (2020): 51, DOI: 10.1080/13697137.2020.1777965; Myra S. Hunter and Joseph Chilcot, "Is Cognitive Behavioral Therapy an Effective Option for Women Who Have Troublesome Menopausal Symptoms?," *British Journal of Health Psychology* 8, no. 26 (2021): 697–708, DOI: 10.1111/bjhp.12543; Sheryl M. Green et al., "Cognitive Behavior Therapy for Menopausal Symptoms (CBT-Meno): A Randomized Controlled Trial," *Menopause* 26, no. 9 (2019): 972–80, DOI: 10.1097/GME.0000000000001363.

64   See, e.g.: Melissa Conklin and Nanette Santoro, "Neurokinin Receptor Antagonists as Potential Nonhormone Treatments for Vasomotor Symptoms," *Therapeutic Advances in Reproductive Health* 17 (2023): 1, DOI: 10.1177/26334941231177611.

65   Aubrey, "Hormones for Menopause Are Safe, Study Finds."

66 See, e.g.: Manson et al., "Menopausal Hormone Therapy and Health Outcomes"; Yoav Arnson et al., "Hormone Replacement Therapy Is Associated with Less Coronary Atherosclerosis and Lower Mortality," *Journal of the American College of Cardiology* 69, no. 11 (2017): 1408, DOI: 10.1016/s0735-1097(17)34797-6; Howard N. Hodis and Wendy J. Mack, "Menopausal Hormone Replacement Therapy and Reduction of All-Cause Mortality and Cardiovascular Disease," *The Cancer Journal* 28, no. 3 (2022): 208, DOI: 10.1097/PPO.0000000000000591; "New Meta-Analysis Shows That Hormone Therapy Can Significantly Reduce Insulin Resistance," The Menopause Society, September 3, 2024, https://menopause.org/press-releases/new-meta-analysis-shows-that-hormone-therapy-can-significantly-reduce-insulin-resistance.

67 Gina Price Lundberg and Nanette Kass Wengr, "Menopause Hormone Therapy: What a Cardiologist Needs to Know," *American College of Cardiology*, July 18, 2019, https://www.acc.org/Latest-in-Cardiology/Articles/2019/07/17/11/56/Menopause-Hormone-Therapy.

68 Samar R. El Khoudary et al., "Menopause Transition and Cardiovascular Disease Risk: Implications for Timing of Early Prevention: A Scientific Statement from the American Heart Association," *Circulation* 142, no. 25 (2020): e506, DOI: 10.1161/CIR.0000000000000912.

69 See, e.g.: "About Women and Heart Disease," Centers for Disease Control and Prevention, accessed October 4, 2024, https://www.cdc.gov/heart-disease/about/women-and-heart-disease.html.

70 C. Z. Zalenga et al., "Association Between the Route of Administration and Formulation of Estrogen Therapy and Hypertension Risk in Postmenopausal Women: A Prospective Population-Based Study," *Hypertension* 80, no. 7 (2023): 1463, DOI: 10.1161HYPERTENSIONAHA.122.19938.

71 Learn more: "Hormone Therapy for Breast Cancer Fact Sheet," *National Cancer Institute*, accessed October 4, 2024, https://www.cancer.gov/types/breast/breast-hormone-therapy-fact-sheet.

72 Wendy Y. Chen and Avrun Bluming, "Counterpoints—Does Combination Menopausal Hormone Therapy Increase the Risk of Breast Cancer? No, Combination MHT Does Not Increase the Risk of Breast Cancer," *Clinical Advances in Hematology & Oncology* 22, no. 9 (2024): 433, https://www.hematologyandoncology.net/archives/november-2024

/does-combination-menopausal-hormone-therapy-increase-the-risk-of-breast-cancer.

73 Spencer Smith, "'Blind Spots' with Dr. Marty Makary," *Self-Funded with Spencer*, September 20, 2024, https://creators.spotify.com/pod/show/spencer-harlan-smith/episodes/Blind-Spots-with-Dr--Marty-Makary-e2oc4hk/a-abhbm7r.

74 Marlene Cimons, "No Need to Fear Menopause Hormone Drugs, Finds Major Women's Health Study," *The Washington Post*, May 1, 2024, https://www.washingtonpost.com/wellness/2024/05/01/menopause-hormones-hrt-safety-whi.

75 A. K. Sinno et al., "Hormone Therapy (HT) in Women with Gynecologic Cancers and in Women at High Risk for Developing a Gynecologic Cancer: A Society of Gynecologic Oncology (SGO) Clinical Practice Statement," *Gynecologic Oncology* 157, no. 2 (2020): 303–6, DOI: 10.1016/j.ygyno.2020.01.035.

76 Jamie DePolo, "Menopause and Menopause Symptoms," Breastcancer.org, June 4, 2024, https://www.breastcancer.org/treatment-side-effects/menopause.

77 Faubion et al., "The 2022 Hormone Therapy Position Statement."

78 Meg Henze and Bronwyn G. A. Stuckey, "Endocrine Consequences of Breast Cancer Therapy and Survivorship," *Climacteric* 27, no. 4 (2024): 333, DOI: 10.1080/13697137.2024.2354725.

79 See also: Cagnacci and Venier, "The Controversial History of Hormone Replacement Therapy."

80 See, e.g.: Gail A. Greendale et al., "Perimenopause and Cognition," *Obstetrics and Gynecology Clinics of North America* 38, no. 3 (2011): 519–35, DOI: 10.1016/j.ogc.2011.05.007; Lisa Mosconi et al., "In Vivo Brain Estrogen Receptor Density by Neuroendocrine Aging and Relationships with Cognition and Symptomatology," *Scientific Reports* 14, no. 1 (2024), DOI: 10.1038/s41598-024-62820-7.

81 Yufan Liu and Chenglong Li, "Hormone Therapy and Biological Aging in Postmenopausal Women," *The Journal of the American Medical Association Network Open* 7, no. 8 (2024), DOI: 10.1001/jamanetworkopen.2024.30839.

82 Jacqueline B. Vo et al., "Trends in Heart Disease Mortality Among Breast Cancer Survivors in the US, 1975–2017," *Breast Cancer Research*

and Treatment 192, no. 3 (2022): 611–22, DOI: 10.1007/s10549-022-06515-5

83   J. A. Cauley et al., "Incidence of Fractures Compared to Cardiovascular Disease and Breast Cancer: The Women's Health Initiative Observational Study," *Osteoporosis International* 19, no. 12 (2008): 1717–23, DOI: 1717–23; 10.1007/s00198-008-0634-y.

84   See, e.g.: "Dr. Kristi Though DeSapri: Bone Health Updates Part 2," *Women's Health by Heather Hirsch*, May 26, 2021, https://heatherhirschmd.com/podcast/86-bone-health-updates-part-2-with-dr-kristi-though-desapri-md/; Veronika A. Levin et al., "Estrogen Therapy for Osteoporosis in the Modern Era," *Osteoporosis International* 29 (2018): 1049, DOI: 10.1007/s00198-018-4414-z.

85   See, e.g.: Sasha Taylor and Susan R. Davis, "Is It Time to Revisit the Recommendations for Initiation of Menopausal Hormone Therapy?" *The Lancet Diabetes & Endocrinology* 13, no. 1 (2024): 69–74, DOI: 10.1016/S2213-8587(24)00270-5.

86   Dominus, "Women Have Been Misled about Menopause."

87   Hannah Wrathall, "How to Rewrite the Anxious Millennopause," Wrapp Consulting, accessed November 3, 2024, https://wrappconsulting.co.uk/wp-content/uploads/2024/08/FINAL-Anxious-Millennopause.pdf.

88   See, e.g.: M. Kathryn Dahlgren et al., "A Survey of Medical Cannabis Use During Perimenopause and Post-Menopause," *Menopause* 29, no. 9 (2022): 1028, DOI: 10.1097/GME.0000000000002018; Maureen Salamon, "Are Women Turning to Cannabis for Menopause Symptom Relief?," Harvard Health Publishing, October 27, 2022, https://www.health.harvard.edu/blog/are-women-turning-to-cannabis-for-menopause-symptom-relief-202210242837; Katherine Babyn et al., "Women's Perceptions and Experiences with Cannabis Use in Menopause: A Qualitative Study," *Menopause* 31, no. 9 (2024): 781–88, DOI: 10.1097/GME.0000000000002388.

Chapter 7

89   Molly Triffin, "Pink Tax: Women Charged More for Beauty Products and Clothes," *Time*, March 4, 2016, https://time.com/4245619/pink-tax-study, citing Department of Consumer Affairs, "From Cradle to Cane: The Cost of Being a Female Consumer," NYC Consumer

Affairs, December 2015, https://www.nyc.gov/assets/dca/downloads/pdf/partners/Study-of-Gender-Pricing-in-NYC.pdf.

90 Department of Consumer Affairs, "From Cradle to Cane."

91 Rakesh Kochhar, "The Enduring Grip of the Gender Pay Gap," Pew Research Center, March 1, 2023, https://www.pewresearch.org/social-trends/2023/03/01/the-enduring-grip-of-the-gender-pay-gap.

92 "What's the Wage Gap in the States?," National Partnership for Women & Families, March 2024, https://nationalpartnership.org/report/wage-gap.

93 "The Motherhood Penalty," AAUW.org, accessed October 14, 2024, https://www.aauw.org/issues/equity/motherhood.

94 "Should Tampons Be Free: Why Are Feminine Products So Expensive?" FSAstore.com, accessed October 15, 2024, https://fsastore.com/articles/learn-tampons-expensive.html.

95 Jessica Kane, "This Is the Price of Your Period," *HuffPost*, last updated December 6, 2017, https://www.huffpost.com/entry/period-cost-lifetime_n_7258780.

96 National Organization for Women, "Female Homelessness and Period Poverty—National Organization for Women," January 22, 2021, https://now.org/blog/female-homelessness-and-period-poverty.

97 Natasha Khan, "Higher Prices on Tampons, Pads Prompt Hard Choices for Americans," *The Wall Street Journal*, July 22, 2024, https://www.wsj.com/business/tampons-pads-price-hikes-de3f3045.

98 "State of the Period 2023," PERIOD.org, accessed October 15, 2024, https://period.org/uploads/2023-State-of-the-Period-Study.pdf.

99 Erika Edwards, "1 in 3 Teens Can't Get Tampons or Pads During Their Periods, Study Finds," *NBC News*, September 26, 2024, https://www.nbcnews.com/health/health-news/1-3-teens-cant-get-tampons-pads-periods-study-finds-rcna172265.

100 "Healthy Habits: Menstrual Hygiene," Centers for Disease Control and Prevention, accessed October 15, 2024, https://www.cdc.gov/hygiene/about/menstrual-hygiene.html.

101 Hafiz Jaafar et al., "Period Poverty: A Neglected Public Health Issue," *Korean Journal of Family Medicine* 44, no. 4 (2023): 183–88, DOI: 10.4082/kjfm.22.0206.

102 "The Facts on Tampons-and How to Use Them Safely," US Food and Drug Administration, accessed October 15, 2024, https://www.fda

.gov/consumers/consumer-updates/facts-tampons-and-how-use-them-safely.

103   Jenni A. Shearston et al., "Tampons as a Source of Exposure to Metal(Loid)s," *Environment International* 190 (2024): 108849, DOI: 10.1016/j.envint.2024.108849.

104   Allison McCann and Amy Schoenfeld Walker, "Abortion Bans Across the Country," *The New York Times*, January 6, 2025, https://www.nytimes.com/interactive/2024/us/abortion-laws-roe-v-wade.html.

105   A. Adler, et al., "Changes in the Frequency and Type of Barriers to Reproductive Health Care Between 2017 and 2021," *JAMA Network Open* 6, no. 4 (2023): e237461, DOI: 10.1001/jamanetworkopen.2023.7461; Gabriela Weigel and Alina Salganicoff, "Potential Impacts of Delaying 'Non-Essential' Reproductive Health Care," Kaiser Family Foundation, June 24, 2020, https://www.kff.org/womens-health-policy/issue-brief/potential-impacts-of-delaying-non-essential-reproductive-health-care.

106   Katie Delach, "The New Midlife: Why 60 Is the New 40," Penn Medicine News, September 7, 2017, https://www.pennmedicine.org/news/news-blog/2017/september/the-new-midlife-why-60-isthe-new-40.

107   "New Center for Sexual Medicine and Menopause Opens," Northwestern Medicine Newsroom; "First of Its Kind Sexual Medicine and Menopause Center Opens at Northwestern," *CBS News*; Wolff, "What Doctors Don't Know About Menopause."

108   Nanette Santoro, "Masters of the Menstrual Cycle or Masters of the Life Cycle?," *Fertility and Sterility* 121, no. 2 (2024): 212, DOI: 10.1016/j.fertnstert.2023.11.017.

109   See, e.g.: Kling et al., "Menopause Management Knowledge in Postgraduate Family Medicine"; Allen et al., "Needs Assessment of Menopause Education."

110   See, e.g.: Cynthia A. Stuenkel et al., "Menopause Step-by-Step, a New Monthly Menopause Education Feature," *Menopause* 31, no. 9 (2024): 737, DOI: 10.1097/gme.0000000000002417; Stuenkel, "What Is Menopause?"

111   "US Attitudes Towards the Availability of Menstrual Supplies in Public Schools and Public Universities," Alliance for Period Supplies, accessed October 15, 2024, https://allianceforperiodsupplies.org/news-releases.

112   "Period Products in Schools," Alliance for Period Supplies, accessed October 15, 2024, https://allianceforperiodsupplies.org/period-products-in-schools.

113   Aimee Picchi, "Gov. Tim Walz Made Tampons Free in Minnesota Schools. Here's Why It's Drawing Trump's Ire," *CBS News*, last updated August 8, 2024, https://www.cbsnews.com/news/tampon-tim-walz-minnesota-law-schools-bathrooms-period-poverty.

114   Jeff Edwards, "New NY Law Tackling 'Period Poverty' Motivated by Scarsdale Sisters," *Patch*, last updated August 29, 2024, https://patch.com/new-york/scarsdale/new-ny-law-tackling-period-poverty-motivated-scarsdale-sisters.

115   Maya Davis, "Getting an IUD Can Hurt. New Guidelines Say Doctors Should Help Patients Manage the Pain," *CNN*, last updated August 10, 2024, https://www.cnn.com/2024/08/10/health/iud-pain-cdc-guidelines-wellness/index.html.

116   "Fact Sheet: President Biden Issues Executive Order and Announces New Actions to Advance Women's Health Research and Innovation," The White House, March 18, 2024, https://www.whitehouse.gov/briefing-room/statements-releases/2024/03/18/fact-sheet-president-biden-issues-executive-order-and-announces-new-actions-to-advance-womens-health-research-and-innovation.

117   See, e.g.: Associated Press, "Jill Biden Reveals $500 Million Plan That Focuses on Women's Health at Clinton Global Initiative," Voice of America, September 23, 2024, https://www.voanews.com/a/jill-biden-reveals-500-million-plan-that-focuses-on-women-s-health-at-clinton-global-initiative/7795502.html.

118   Sarah M. Temkin et al., "Perspectives from Advancing National Institutes of Health Research to Inform and Improve the Health of Women," *Obstetrics & Gynecology* 140, no. 1 (2022): 10. DOI: 10.1097/AOG.0000000000004821.

119   Regina Schaffer, "Hormone Therapy Use Among Menopausal Women Continues to Decline, Despite Proven Safety," *Healio*, September 13, 2024, https://www.healio.com/news/womens-health-ob-gyn/20240913/hormone-therapy-use-among-menopausal-women-continues-to-decline-despite-proven-safety.

120   "A Collective of Independent Programs Joined Together to Address Period Poverty in Local Communities in the US," Alliance

for Period Supplies, last accessed February 24, 2025, https://allianceforperiodsupplies.org/allied-programs.

Chapter 8

121 See, e.g.: Sandy Cohen, "Treating the Mental Health Side of Menopause," *UCLA Health*, October 24, 2023, https://www.uclahealth.org/news/article/treating-mental-health-side-menopause.

122 "Women and Anxiety," US Food & Drug Administration, accessed October 15, 2024, https://www.fda.gov/consumers/womens-health-topics/women-and-anxiety.

123 Jake M. Najman et al., "Does the Millennial Generation of Women Experience More Mental Illness Than Their Mothers?" *BMC Psychiatry* 21, no. 1 (2021), DOI: 10.1186/s12888-021-03361-5.

124 "The State of Women… Isn't Working," theSkimm, March 9, 2023, https://www.theskimm.com/stateofwomen/harris-poll-data-2023.

125 Hannah Seligson, "Being a Mother Is Hard Work. Is It Actually Harder on Millennial Moms?" *The New York Times*, May 11, 2024, https://www.nytimes.com/2024/05/11/style/millennial-mom-midlife-crisis.html; Stephanie Hallett, "Millennial Moms Don't Have It All, They Just Do It All," *HuffPost*, last updated June 10, 2024, https://www.huffpost.com/entry/millennial-moms-dont-have-it-all-they-just-do-it-all_1_6660b693e4b06a0c0d1f952b.

126 Kaitlin Grelle, "The Generation Gap Revisited: Generational Differences in Mental Health, Maladaptive Coping Behaviors, and Pandemic-Related Concerns During the Initial COVID-19 Pandemic," *Journal of Adult Development* 16, no. 1 (2023): 1, DOI: 10.1007/s10804-023-09442-x.

127 Sara Srygley et al., "Losing More Ground: Revisiting Young Women's Well-being Across Generations," *Population Bulletin* 77, no. 1 (2023), https://www.prb.org/wp-content/uploads/2023/11/Losing-More-Ground_Population-Bulletin-Vol-77-No-1.pdf.

128 See also: Aljumah Rawan et al., "An Online Survey of Postmenopausal Women to Determine Their Attitudes and Knowledge of the Menopause," *Post Reproductive Health* 29, no. 2 (2023): 67, DOI: 10.1177/20533691231166543.

129 See, e.g.: Santoro, "Menopause Step-by-Step"; Ellen W. Freeman, "Associations of Depression with the Transition to Menopause," *Menopause* 17, no. 4 (2010): 823, DOI: 10.1097/gme.0b013e3181db9f8b.

130   "Mental Health," The Menopause Society, accessed October 15, 2024, https://menopause.org/patient-education/menopause-topics/mental-health. See also: Ellen W. Freeman, "Depression in the Menopause Transition: Risks in the Changing Hormone Milieu as Observed in the General Population," *Women's Midlife Health* 1, no. 2 (2015), DOI: 10.1186/s40695-015-0002-y.

131   Joyce T. Bromberger, "Major Depression During and After the Menopausal Transition: Study of Women's Health Across the Nation (SWAN)," *Psychological Medicine* 41, no. 9 (2011): 1879, DOI:10.1017/S003329171100016X; Samar R. El Khoudary et al., "The Menopause Transition and Women's Health at Midlife: A Progress Report from the Study of Women's Health Across The Nation (SWAN)," *Menopause* 26, no. 10 (2019): 1213, DOI: 10.1097/GME.0000000000001424; Joyce T. Bromberger and Cynthia Neill Epperson, "Depression During and After the Perimenopause," *Obstetrics and Gynecology Clinics of North America* 45, no. 4 (2018): 663, DOI: 10.1016/j.ogc.2018.07.007. See also: Yasmee Badawy et al., "The Risk of Depression in the Menopausal Stages: A Systematic Review And Meta-Analysis," *Journal of Affective Disorders* 357 (2024): 126, DOI: 10.1016/j.jad.2024.04.041.

132   See, e.g.: Lydia Brown and Martha Hickey, "The Course of Depressive Symptoms over Midlife," *Menopause* 31, no. 12 (2024): 1033, DOI: 10.1097/GME.0000000000002464; Diana Chirinos et al., "Trajectories of Depressive Symptoms in a Population-Based Cohort of Black and White Women from Late Reproductive Age Through the Menopause Transition: A 30-Year Analysis," *Menopause* 31, no. 12 (2024): 1035, DOI: 10.1097/GME.0000000000002447.

133   Freeman, "Associations of Depression with the Transition to Menopause."

134   See, e.g.: Suna Huang et al., "Anxiety Disorder in Menopausal Women and the Intervention Efficacy of Mindfulness-Based Stress Reduction," *American Journal of Translational Research* 15, no. 3 (2023): 2016, PMID: 37056841; Marianna de Jaeger et al., "Negative Affect Symptoms, Anxiety Sensitivity, and Vasomotor Symptoms During Perimenopause," *Brazilian Journal of Psychiatry* 43, no. 3 (2021): 277, DOI: 10.1590/1516-4446-2020-0871; Joyce Bromberger et al., "Does Risk for Anxiety Increase During the Menopausal Transition? Study of Women's Health Across the Nation," *Menopause* 20, no. 5 (2013): 488, DOI: 10.1097/GME.0b013e3182730599.

135 See, e.g.: Jayashri Kulkarni, "Perimenopausal Depression—an Under-Recognized Entity," *Australian Prescriber* 41, no. 6 (2018): 183, DOI: 10.18773/austprescr.2018.060; Miharu Nakanishi et al., "Association Between Menopause and Suicidal Ideation in Mothers of Adolescents: A Longitudinal Study Using Data from a Population-Based Cohort," *Journal of Affective Disorders* 340 (2023): 529, DOI: 10.1016/j.jad.2023.08.055; "Suicidality in Midlife Women: A Brief Overview," MGH Center for Women's Mental Health, September 24, 2020, https://womensmentalhealth.org/posts/suicidality-midlife/; "My Story: Losing My Wife—an Avoidable Tragedy?" balance by Newson Health, March 8, 2022, https://www.balance-menopause.com/menopause-library/my-story-losing-my-wife-an-avoidable-tragedy..

136 Salama Alblooshi et al., "Does Menopause Elevate the Risk for Developing Depression and Anxiety? Results from a Systematic Review," *Australasian Psychiatry* 31, no. 2 (2023): 165, DOI: 10.1177/10398562231165439.

137 Claudio Soares, "Depression in Peri- and Postmenopausal Women: Prevalence, Pathophysiology and Pharmacological Management," *Drugs & Aging* 30, no. 9 (2013): 677, DOI: 10.1007/s40266-013-0100-1.

138 Anita Clayton and Philip T. Nanin, "Depression or Menopause? Presentation and Management of Major Depressive Disorder in Perimenopausal and Postmenopausal Women," *Primary Care Companion to The Journal of Clinical Psychiatry* 12, no. 1 (2010), DOI: 10.4088/PCC.08r00747blu.

139 Yuefang Chang, "Lifetime History of Depression and Anxiety Disorders as a Predictor of Quality of Life in Midlife Women in the Absence of Current Illness Episodes," *Archives of General Psychiatry* 69, no. 5 (2012): 484, DOI: 10.1001/archgenpsychiatry.2011.1578.

140 "Menopause and Mental Health," Harvard Health Publishing of Harvard Medical School, March 1, 2020, https://www.health.harvard.edu/womens-health/menopause-and-mental-health.

141 Tori DeAngelis, "Menopause Can Be Rough. Psychology Is Here to Help," *Monitor on Psychology* 54, no. 6 (2023), https://www.apa.org/monitor/2023/09/easing-transition-into-menopause.

142 Nazanin E. Silver, "Mood Changes During Perimenopause Are Real. Here's What to Know," *The American College of Obstetricians and Gynecologists*, April 2023, https://www.acog.org/womens-health/experts

-and-stories/the-latest/mood-changes-during-perimenopause-are-real-heres-what-to-know.

143   Nina Coslov, "'Not Feeling like Myself' in Perimenopause—What Does It Mean? Observations from the Women Living Better Survey," *Menopause* 31, no. 5 (2024): 390, DOI: 10.1097/GME.0000000000002339.

144   Lisa Shitomi-Jones et al., "Exploration of First Onsets of Mania, Schizophrenia Spectrum Disorders and Major Depressive Disorder in Perimenopause," *Nature Mental Health* 2 (2024): 1161, DOI: 10.1038/s44220-024-00292-4.

145   See, e.g.: Cohen, "Treating the Mental Health Side of Menopause"; "Hormones & Mental Health: Understanding Perimenopause and Beyond with Dr. Suzanne Fenske," *Alluminate with Dr. Allie Sharma Podcast*, February 12, 2025, https://alluminate-with-dr-allie-sharma.simplecast.com/episodes/hormones-mental-health-understanding-perimenopause-and-beyond-with-dr-suzanne-fenske-3My2kAg9.

146   DeAngelis, "Menopause Can Be Rough."

147   Silver, "Mood Changes During Perimenopause Are Real. Here's What to Know."

148   See, e.g.: Sonali Lokuge et al., "The Rapid Effects of Estrogen: A Mini-Review," *Behavioural Pharmacology* 21, nos. 5–6 (2010): 465, DOI: 10.1097/FBP.0b013e32833da5c3; Daniella Swales et al., "Hormone Sensitivity Predicts the Beneficial Effects of Transdermal Estradiol on Reward-Seeking Behaviors in Perimenopausal Women: A Randomized Controlled Trial," *Psychoneuroendocrinology* 156 (2023), DOI: 10.1016/j.psyneuen.2023.106339 10.1016/j.psyneuen.2023.106339.

149   Claudio Soares et al., "Efficacy of Estradiol for the Treatment of Depressive Disorders in Perimenopausal Women: A Double-Blind, Randomized, Placebo-Controlled Trial," *Archives of General Psychiatry* 58, no. 6 (2001): 529, DOI: 10.1001/archpsyc.58.6.529.

150   Alblooshi, "Does Menopause Elevate the Risk for Developing Depression and Anxiety?"

151   Alblooshi, "Does Menopause Elevate the Risk for Developing Depression and Anxiety?"

152   Hunter, "Cognitive Behavioral Therapy for Menopause Symptoms."

153   Hunter, "Cognitive Behavioral Therapy for Menopause Symptoms"; Cohen, "Treating the Mental Health Side of Menopause."

154 See, e.g.: Jayashri Kulkarni et al., "Development and Validation of a New Rating Scale for Perimenopausal Depression—The Meno-D," *Translational Psychiatry* 8, no. 123 (2018), DOI: 10.1038/s41398-018-0172-0.

155 See, e.g.: Subhadra Evans et al., "The Need for Biopsychosocial Menopause Care: A Narrative Review," *Menopause* 31, no. 12 (2024): 1090, DOI: 10.1097/GME.0000000000002441.

156 Jie Wen et al., "The Psychological Side of Menopause: Evidence from the Comorbidity Network Of Menopausal, Anxiety, and Depressive Symptoms," *Menopause* 31, no. 10 (2024): 897, DOI: 10.1097/GME.0000000000002406.

157 Cecilia Tasca, "Women and Hysteria in the History of Mental Health," *Clinical Practice & Epidemiology in Mental Health* 8, no. 1 (2012): 110, DOI: 10.2174/1745017901208010110.

Chapter 9

158 See, e.g.: Gail Greendale et al., "Perimenopause and Cognition," *Obstetrics and Gynecology Clinics of North America* 38, no. 3 (2011): 519, DOI: 10.1016/j.ogc.2011.05.007; Kunihiko Hayashi et al., "Complaints of Reduced Cognitive Functioning During Perimenopause: A Cross-Sectional Analysis of the Japan Nurses' Health Study," *Women's Midlife Health* 8, no. 1 (2022), DOI: 10.1186/s40695-022-00076-9.

159 Michelina McCarthy and Ami P. Raval, "The Peri-Menopause in a Woman's Life: A Systemic Inflammatory Phase That Enables Later Neurodegenerative Disease," *Journal of Neuroinflammation* 17, no. 317 (2020), DOI: 10.1186/s12974-020-01998-9.

160 See, e.g.: Jim Sliwinski et al., "Memory Decline in Peri- and Post-Menopausal Women: The Potential of Mind–Body Medicine to Improve Cognitive Performance," *Integrative Medicine Insights* 9 (2014), DOI: 10.4137/IMI.S15682.

161 Katie Hawkins-Gaar, "'Mommy Brain' Is Real," *The New York Times*, July 14, 2021, https://www.nytimes.com/2021/07/14/parenting/mom-brain-forgetfulness-science.html.

162 Laura DeFina et al., "The Association Between Midlife Cardiorespiratory Fitness Levels and Later-Life Dementia," *Annals of Internal Medicine* 158, no. 3 (2013): 162, DOI: 10.7326/0003-4819-158-3-201302050-00005; Helena Hörder et al., "Midlife Cardiovascular

Fitness and Dementia," *Neurology* 90, no. 15 (2018): e1298, DOI: 10.1212/WNL.0000000000005290.

163 See, e.g.: Joan Lo et al., "Bone and the Perimenopause," *Obstetrics and Gynecology Clinics of North America* 38, no. 3 (2011): 503, DOI: 10.1016/j.ogc.2011.07.001.

164 "What Women Need to Know," Bone Health & Osteoporosis Foundation, accessed October 15, 2024, https://www.bonehealthandosteoporosis.org/preventing-fractures/general-facts/what-women-need-to-know.

165 See also: Eliza Barclay, "No One Told Me This Would Happen to My Body in My 40s," *The New York Times*, October 27, 2024, https://www.nytimes.com/2024/10/27/opinion/body-muscles-40s-aging.html.

166 Vonda Wright, "The Musculoskeletal Syndrome of Menopause," *Climacteric* 27, no. 5 (2024): 466, DOI: 10.1080/13697137.2024.2380363. See also: Danielle Friedman, "Has Menopause Made You Ache All Over? There's a Name for That," *The New York Times*, November 20, 2024, https://www.nytimes.com/2024/11/20/well/move/menopause-muscle-pain-body-aches.html.

167 See, e.g.: "Mediterranean Diet for Heart Health," *Mayo Clinic*, July 15, 2023, https://www.mayoclinic.org/healthy-lifestyle/nutrition-and-healthy-eating/in-depth/mediterranean-diet/art-20047801; Elke Trautwein and Sue McKay, "The Role of Specific Components of a Plant-Based Diet in Management of Dyslipidemia and the Impact on Cardiovascular Risk," *Nutrients* 12, no. 9 (2020): 2671, DOI: 10.3390/nu12092671.

168 Juliana Kling et al., "Associations of Sleep and Female Sexual Function: Good Sleep Quality Matters," *Menopause* 28, no. 6 (2021): 619, DOI: 10.1097/gme.0000000000001744.

169 Damien Léger et al., "'You Look Sleepy…' the Impact of Sleep Restriction on Skin Parameters and Facial Appearance of 24 Women," *Sleep Medicine* 89 (2022): 97, DOI: 10.1016/j.sleep.2021.11.011.

170 P. Oyetakin-White et al., "Does Poor Sleep Quality Affect Skin Ageing?," *Clinical and Experimental Dermatology* 40, no. 1 (2015): 17, DOI: 10.1111/ced.12455.

171 See, e.g.: Zhang Feng and Long Cheng, "Association Between Sleep Duration and Depression in Menopausal Women: A Population-Based Study," *Frontiers in Endocrinology* 15 (2024), DOI: 10.3389

/fendo.2024.1301775; Silver, "Mood Changes During Perimenopause Are Real."

172   See, e.g.: Karin Frank-Raue and Friedhelm Raue, "Thyroid Dysfunction in Peri- and Postmenopausal Women—Cumulative Risks," *Deutsches Ärzteblatt International* 120, no. 18 (2023): 311, DOI: 10.3238/arztebl.m2023.0069; Manjusha Yadav et al., "Frequency of Thyroid Disorder in Pre- and Postmenopausal Women and Its Association with Menopause Symptoms," *Cureus* 15, no. 6 (2023), DOI: 10.7759/cureus.e40900.

173   See also: Cormac Kennedy et al., "The Effect of Semaglutide on Blood Pressure in Patients Without Diabetes: A Systematic Review and Meta-Analysis," *Journal of Clinical Medicine* 12, no. 3 (2023): 772, DOI: 10.3390/jcm12030772; Maria Hurtado et al., "Weight Loss Response to Semaglutide in Postmenopausal Women with and Without Hormone Therapy Use," *Menopause* 31, no. 4 (2024): 266, DOI: 10.1097/GME.0000000000002310.

174   See, e.g.: Mateusz Kozinoga et al., "Low Back Pain in Women Before and After Menopause," *Menopausal Review* 14, no. 3 (2015): 203, DOI: 10.5114/pm.2015.54347.

Chapter 10

175   See, e.g.: "Sexual Health," The Menopause Society, accessed October 17, 2024, https://menopause.org/patient-education/menopause-topics/sexual-health; Holly Thomas et al., "'I Want to Feel like I Used to Feel': A Qualitative Study of Causes of Low Libido in Postmenopausal Women," *Menopause* 27, no. 3 (2020): 289, DOI: 10.1097/gme.0000000000001455; Holly Thomas et al., "Female Sexual Function at Midlife and Beyond," *Obstetrics and Gynecology Clinics of North America* 45, no. 4 (2018): 709, DOI: 10.1016/j.ogc.2018.07.013.

176   Kelli Stidham Hall et al., "Stress Symptoms and Frequency of Sexual Intercourse Among Young Women," *The Journal of Sexual Medicine* 11, no. 8 (2014): 1982, DOI: 10.1111/jsm.12607.

177   "New Research Reveals Major Gaps and New Solutions in Menopause Care," Kinsey Institute at Indiana University, September 16, 2024, https://kinseyinstitute.org/news-events/news/2024-09-16-menopause.php.

178   Kling, "Associations of Sleep and Female Sexual Function."

179   Emily Harris et al., "Gender Inequities in Household Labor Predict Lower Sexual Desire in Women Partnered with Men," *Archives of Sexual Behavior* 51, no. 8 (2022): 3847, DOI: 10.1007/s10508-022-02397-2; E. Aviv, et al., "Cognitive Household Labor: Gender Disparities and Consequences for Maternal Mental Health and Wellbeing," *Archives of Women's Mental Health* 28 (2025): 5, DOI: 10.1007/s00737-024-01490-w.

180   Sharon Parish et al., "International Society for the Study of Women's Sexual Health Clinical Practice Guideline for the Use of Systemic Testosterone for Hypoactive Sexual Desire Disorder in Women," *The Journal of Sexual Medicine* 18, no. 5 (2021): 849, DOI: 10.1016/j.jsxm.2020.10.009.

181   Sarah Glynne et al., "Effect of Transdermal Testosterone Therapy on Mood and Cognitive Symptoms in Peri- and Postmenopausal Women: A Pilot Study," *Archives of Women's Mental Health* (2024), DOI: 10.1007/s00737-024-01513-6.

182   See, e.g.: E. Stanley, et al., "Gap in Sexual Dysfunction Management Between Male and Female Patients Seen in Primary Care: An Observational Study," *Journal of General Internal Medicine* 40 (2025): 845, DOI: DOI: 10.1007/s11606-024-09004-1.

183   D. Dillo, "I Tried Addyi, the Sex Pill for Women—and Here's What Happened in My Marriage (Exclusive)," *People*, July 1, 2024, https://people.com/addyi-little-pink-pill-women-low-sex-drive-exclusive-8671806.

Chapter 11

184   C. Abraham, "An OB-GYN's Top Tips for Managing Hot Flashes," *The American College of Obstetricians and Gynecologists*, August 2023, https://www.acog.org/womens-health/experts-and-stories/the-latest/an-ob-gyns-top-tips-for-managing-hot-flashes.

185   Alana Semuels, "More U.S. Companies Are Starting to Talk about Menopause," *Time*, June 29, 2023, https://time.com/6290706/menopause-care-work-us-companies.

186   "Menopause in the Workplace Report 2022," Elektra Health, July 11, 2022, https://www.elektrahealth.com/workplacemenopausesurvey.

187   "Break Through the Stigma: Menopause in the Workplace," Bank of America, August 2024, https://business.bofa.com/content/dam/flagship/workplace-benefits/id20_0905/documents/BofA_Lifestage-Report.pdf.

188 "Unveiling the Impact of Menopause in the Workplace," Korn Ferry, August 3, 2023, https://www.kornferry.com/institute/korn-ferry-and-vira-health-survey-findings.

189 "Break Through the Stigma: Menopause in the Workplace," Bank of America. See, also: J. Sauer, "'Powering Through' Is Not Enough," *AARP*, April 25, 2024, DOI: 10.26419/res.00720.008.

190 See, e.g.: "'Millenopause': How HR Leaders Can Support Millennials Navigating Menopause," Maven, October 1, 2024, https://www.mavenclinic.com/post/millenopause-how-hr-leaders-can-support-millennials-navigating-menopause.

191 C. Ewing and C. Leu, "Employers Are Taking Meaningful Steps to Provide Menopause Benefits," Mercer, October 19, 2023, https://www.mercer.com/en-us/insights/us-health-news/employers-are-taking-meaningful-steps.

192 "The State of Perimenopause in 2024," Oova.

193 C. Munn et al., "Menopause Knowledge and Education in Women under 40: Results from an Online Survey," *Women's Health* (London) 18 (2022), DOI: 10.1177/17455057221139660.

194 "Menopause in the Workplace 2023: A Report from Carrot Fertility," Carrot Fertility, accessed November 1, 2024, https://www.get-carrot.com/blog/menopause-in-the-workplace-2023-a-report-from-carrot-fertility.

195 "Menopause in the Workplace Report 2022," Elektra Health, July 11, 2022, https://www.elektrahealth.com/workplacemenopausesurvey.

196 "Menopause in the Workplace 2023," Carrot Fertility.

197 "Menopause in the Workplace 2023," Carrot Fertility.

198 Alisha Haridasani Gupta, "The Next Frontier for Corporate Benefits: Menopause," *The New York Times*, August 19, 2023, https://www.nytimes.com/2023/08/19/business/corporate-benefits-menopause.html.

199 "Menopause Workplace Pledge," Wellbeing of Women, accessed November 10, 2024, https://www.wellbeingofwomen.org.uk/menopause-workplace-pledge.

200 K. Butler, "Menopause Benefits Are Latest Corporate Perk at Microsoft, Abercrombie and NBA," *Bloomberg*, October 24, 2023, https://www.bloomberg.com/news/articles/2023-10-24/menopause-benefits-are-latest-corporate-perk-at-microsoft-abercrombie-and-nba.

201   K. Butler, "US Millennial Women Willing to Quit Jobs Due to Menopause in Study," *Bloomberg*, September 30, 2024, https://www.bloomberg.com/news/articles/2024-09-30/us-millennial-women-willing-to-quit-jobs-due-to-menopause-in-study.

202   "Breaking the Silence on Menopause," Genentech, October 15, 2024, https://www.gene.com/stories/breaking-the-silence-on-menopause.

203   "Women's Health," Adobe, accessed November 16, 2024, https://benefits.adobe.com/us/health-care/specialty-care/womens-health.

204   "2024 Report: Maven's State of Women's & Family Health Benefits," Maven, accessed November 1, 2024. https://info.mavenclinic.com/pdf/state-women-family-health-benefits-2024.

205   Haridasani Gupta, "The Next Frontier for Corporate Benefits."

206   "Break Through the Stigma: Menopause in the Workplace," Bank of America.

207   See also: National Menopause Foundation, "Workplace Fairness for Women at Midlife: A Conversation on Menopause and Employee Rights," *The Positive Pause Podcast*, October 29, 2024, https://nationalmenopausefoundation.org/episode-28-workplace-fairness-for-women-at-midlife.

208   "Biote Women in the Workplace Survey," Biote, December 1, 2022, https://biote.com/learning-center/biote-women-in-the-workplace-survey.

209   S. Faubion et al., "Impact of Menopause Symptoms on Women in the Workplace," *Mayo Clinic Proceedings* 98, no. 6 (2023): 833, DOI: 10.1016/j.mayocp.2023.02.025.

210   "A Checklist to Help Women Navigate Their Menopause Journey," Bank of America, accessed November 2, 2024, https://nationalmenopausefoundation.org/wp-content/uploads/2023/10/BofA_RRI_Menopause_Checklist_1023_FINAL-MAP-ADA.pdf.

211   "Beyond HRT: Building Better Menopause & Midlife Health Benefits," Maven, accessed November 1, 2024, https://www.mavenclinic.com/resource-hub/beyond-hrt-building-better-menopause-midlife-health-benefits.

212   Rees Margaret et al., "Global Consensus Recommendations on Menopause in the Workplace: A European Menopause and Andropause Society (EMAS) Position Statement," *Maturitas* 151 (2021): 55, DOI: 10.1016/j.maturitas.2021.06.006.

213 "Making Menopause Work," The Menopause Society, September 12, 2024, https://menopause.org/workplace.

214 A. Diehl et al., "Women in Leadership Face Ageism at Every Age," *Harvard Business Review*, June 20, 2023, https://hbr.org/2023/06/women-in-leadership-face-ageism-at-every-age; K. M. Korducki, "A New Study Makes It Official: Women Are Always the Wrong Age for Employers," *Business Insider*, August 2023, https://www.businessinsider.com/discrimination-at-work-women-all-ages-jobs-hiring-employer-bosses-2023-8.

215 S. Krawcheck, "Why Is 'Menopause' a NSFW Word?" LinkedIn, August 10, 2024, https://www.linkedin.com/pulse/why-menopause-nsfw-word-sallie-krawcheck-w5fvc/?trackingId=0Vxfs0ZgRbSCP1oWCMRBEg%3D%3D.

216 M. Travis, "What Employers Should Know About Menopause Discrimination," *Forbes*, June 4, 2024, https://www.forbes.com/sites/michelletravis/2024/05/21/what-employers-should-know-about-menopause-discrimination.

Chapter 12

217 Munn, "Menopause Knowledge and Education."

218 S. Brown and I-Fen Lin, "The Graying of Divorce: A Half Century of Change," *The Journals of Gerontology: Series B* 77, no. 9 (2022): 1710, DOI: 10.1093/geronb/gbac057.

219 See, e.g.: "Menopause Puts Final Nail in Marriage Coffin," balance by Newson Health, October 18, 2022, https://www.balance-menopause.com/news/menopause-puts-final-nail-in-marriage-coffin; R. Hopegood, "Do I Really Want a Divorce? Or Is It Menopause?" *Oprah Daily*, August 15, 2024, https://www.oprahdaily.com/life/health/a61805675/divorce-during-menopause.

220 See, e.g.: R. Fry, "In a Growing Share of US Marriages, Husbands and Wives Earn About the Same," Pew Research Center, April 13, 2023, https://www.pewresearch.org/social-trends/2023/04/13/in-a-growing-share-of-u-s-marriages-husbands-and-wives-earn-about-the-same; Aviv, "Cognitive Household Labor."

221 S. Parish, "The Mate Survey: Men's Perceptions and Attitudes Towards Menopause and Their Role in Partners' Menopausal Transition," *Menopause* 26, no. 10 (2019): 1110, DOI: 10.1097/GME.0000000000001373.

Chapter 13

222   "Menopause Market Size, Share & Trends Analysis Report by Treatment (Dietary Supplements, OTC Pharma Products), by Region (North America, Europe, Latin America), and Segment Forecasts, 2024–2030," Grand View Research, accessed October 17, 2024, https://www.grandviewresearch.com/industry-analysis/menopause-market.

223   "Menopause Market Size to Hit USD 27.63 Billion by 2033," Straits Research, November 21, 2024, https://www.globenewswire.com/news-release/2024/11/21/2985347/0/en/Menopause-Market-Size-to-Hit-USD-27-63-Billion-by-2033-Straits-Research.html.

224   See, e.g.: L. Loacker, "Project W: Pulling Back the Curtain on Menopause," David Wright Tremaine LLP, March 7, 2024, https://www.dwt.com/insights/2024/03/pulling-back-the-curtain-on-menopause.

225   B. Barreto and S. Bhatia, "Menopause," Femhealth Insights, accessed October 17, 2024, https://www.femhealthinsights.com/reports/p/menopause.

226   See, e.g.: C. Hall, "Why More Startups and VCs Are Finally Pursuing the Menopause Market: '$600B Is Not 'Niche,''" *Crunchbase News*, February 14, 2022, https://news.crunchbase.com/startups/menopause-startups-vc-funding; E. Hinchliffe, "Menopause Is a $600 Billion Opportunity, Report Finds," *Fortune*, October 26, 2020, https://fortune.com/2020/10/26/menopause-startups-female-founders-fund-report.

227   J. Sauer, "The Economic Impact of Menopause: A Survey of Women 35+ and Employers," *AARP*, January 2024, DOI: 10.26419/res.00720.001.

228   "Menopause: The $600 Billion Opportunity in Femtech," Prescouter, accessed October 17, 2024, https://www.prescouter.com/inquiry/the-menopause-market-the-600-billion-opportunity-in-femtech.

229   Barreto and Bhatia, "Menopause."

230   See, e.g.: Hinchliffe, "Menopause Is a $600 Billion Opportunity"; "SJF Market Analysis Outlines Startups Disrupting Menopause Care, Opportunities for Investors," *SJF Ventures*, accessed October 17, 2024, https://sjfventures.com/sjf-ventures-market-analysis-outlines-startups-disrupting-menopause-care-and-opportunities-for-investors.

231 Barreto and Bhatia, "Menopause."; See also: D. Shunina, "FemTech Startups' Uphill Battle for Funding," *Forbes*, last updated February 12, 2024, https://www.forbes.com/sites/dariashunina/2024/02/09/femtech-startups-uphill-battle-for-funding.

232 A. Hill, "Women's Health Tech 'Less Likely' to Get Funding If Woman Is on Founding Team," *The Guardian*, October 8, 2024, https://www.theguardian.com/society/2024/oct/08/womens-health-tech-less-likely-to-get-funding-if-woman-is-on-founding-team.

233 See also: H. Lewis, "Capitalism Has Plans for Menopause," *The Atlantic*, October 30, 2023, https://www.theatlantic.com/ideas/archive/2023/10/menopause-activism-influencers-books/675762; E. Burns, "The Hype Is Up: Here Is What Is Really Needed to Drive Sales for Menopause Brands," *Women's Wear Daily*, August 6, 2024, https://wwd.com/beauty-industry-news/wellness/menopause-products-devices-supplements-topicals-1236514547.

234 See, e.g.: L. Taylor-Swanson et al., "Midlife Women's Menopausal Transition Symptom Experience and Access to Medical and Integrative Health Care: Informing the Development of MENOGAP," *Global Advances in Integrative Medicine and Health* 13 (2024), DOI: 10.1177/27536130241268355.

235 See, e.g.: F. Britten, "Do You Need a 'Menopause Doula'?" *The Times*, November 10, 2024, https://www.thetimes.com/life-style/health-fitness/article/menopause-doula-midlife-coach-advice-help-nfcjlrt35.

236 M. Roberts, "HRT Prescriptions in England up 22% in a Year," *BBC*, October 17, 2024, https://www.bbc.com/news/articles/cgj4qp5j197o.

237 "Breaking the Silence: Carolyn Harris MP's Journey and Fight for Menopause Awareness," Chamber UK, August 15, 2024, https://chamberuk.com/fight-for-menopause-awareness.

238 "B.C. Pharmacare Deal Will Cover Diabetes Meds, Hormone Therapy," *The Canadian Press*, September 12, 2024, https://www.cbc.ca/news/canada/british-columbia/b-c-pharmacare-deal-will-cover-diabetes-meds-hormone-therapy-1.7322046.

239 N. Ireland, "How Menopause Awareness Among Employers, Patients Is Changing the Workplace," *The Canadian Press*, November 25, 2024, https://www.ctvnews.ca/health/how-menopause-awareness-among-employers-patients-is-changing-the-workplace-1.7122301.

240   J. Bray, "Free HRT to be Available from Next January Under Cabinet Plans," *Irish Times*, October 15, 2024, https://www.irishtimes.com/health/2024/10/15/free-hrt-to-be-available-from-next-january-under-cabinet-plans.

241   See also: N. Lansen and Jannine Versi, "We Need Better Menopause Care, Especially for Women of Color," *Ms. Magazine*, October 17, 2024, https://msmagazine.com/2024/10/17/we-need-better-menopause-care-especially-for-women-of-color.

242   Learn more: Kim Hart and April Haberman, "Pioneering FemTech and Bridging Gaps in Women's Healthcare with Dr. Brittany Barreto," *The MiDOViA Menopause Podcast*, August 26, 2024, https://podcasts.apple.com/us/podcast/episode-025-pioneering-femtech-and-bridging-gaps-in/id1732534331?i=1000666675311.

Chapter 14

243   See, e.g.: K. Angelou et al., "The Genitourinary Syndrome of Menopause: An Overview of the Recent Data," *Cureus* 12, no. 4 (2020): e7586, DOI: 10.7759/cureus.7586.

244   E. Micks, "Sexually Transmitted Infections in Midlife Women," *Menopause* 31, no. 5 (2024): 430, DOI: 10.1097/GME.0000000000002345.

245   See, e.g.: E. Moral et al., "Genitourinary Syndrome of Menopause. Prevalence and Quality of Life in Spanish Postmenopausal Women, the GENISSE Study," *Climacteric* 21, no. 2 (2018): 167, DOI: 10.1080/13697137.2017.1421921.

246   S. Cichowski, "UTIs after Menopause: Why They're Common and What to Do About Them," *The American College of Obstetrician and Gynecologists*, November 2023, https://www.acog.org/womens-health/experts-and-stories/the-latest/utis-after-menopause-why-theyre-common-and-what-to-do-about-them.

247   Kimberly Peacock et al., *Menopause* (Stat Peals Publishing, 2024), https://www.ncbi.nlm.nih.gov/books/NBK507826.

248   Kozinoga, "Low Back Pain in Women."

249   "Menopause and Bone Loss," Endocrine Society, January 24, 2022, https://www.endocrine.org/patient-engagement/endocrine-library/menopause-and-bone-loss.

250   See, e.g.: N. Reza et al., "Representation of Women in Heart Failure Clinical Trials: Barriers to Enrollment and Strategies to Close the Gap," *American Heart Journal Plus: Cardiology Research and Practice* 13 (2022), DOI: 10.1016/j.ahjo.2022.100093; C. Carland et al., "Adequate Enrollment of Women in Cardiovascular Drug Trials and the Need for Sex-Specific Assessment and Reporting," *American Heart Journal Plus: Cardiology Research and Practice* 17 (2022): 100155, DOI: 10.1016/j.ahjo.2022.100155.

251   See, e.g.: E. Hayward, "Women Die Needlessly as NHS Treats Heart Trouble as a Man's Disease," *The Times*, September 25, 2024, https://www.thetimes.com/uk/healthcare/article/women-die-needlessly-as-nhs-treats-heart-trouble-as-a-mans-disease-gn66dswcj; A. Huebschmann and J. Regensteiner, "The Gender Gap in Heart Disease Research, Treatment Leaves Women Behind," *The Washington Post*, October 20, 2024, https://www.washingtonpost.com/health/2024/10/20/women-heart-disease-stroke-death.

252   "The Facts about Women and Heart Disease," American Heart Association, accessed October 12, 2024, https://www.goredforwomen.org/en/about-heart-disease-in-women/facts.

253   See, e.g.: K. Ryczkowska et al., "Menopause and Women's Cardiovascular Health: Is It Really an Obvious Relationship?," *Archives of Medical Science* 19, no. 2 (2022): 458, DOI: 10.5114/aoms/157308; H. Currie and Christine Williams, "Menopause, Cholesterol and Cardiovascular Disease," *US Cardiology* 5, no. 1 (2008): 12, DOI: 10.15420/usc.2008.5.1.12.

254   E. Barinas-Mitchell et al., "Cardiovascular Disease Risk Factor Burden During the Menopause Transition and Late Midlife Subclinical Vascular Disease: Does Race/Ethnicity Matter?," *Journal of the American Heart Association* 9, no. 4 (2020), DOI: 10.1161/JAHA.119.013876.

255   El Khoudary, "Menopause Transition and Cardiovascular Disease Risk."

256   A. Calle et al., "Severe Menopause Symptoms Linked to Cognitive Impairment: An Exploratory Study," *Menopause* 31, no. 11 (2024): 959, DOI: 10.1097/GME.0000000000002422.

257   Greendale et al., "Perimenopause and Cognition."

258   See, e.g.: Greendale, "Perimenopause and Cognition"; "Heart Disease Linked to Dementia in Women," American Heart Association,

December 7, 2023, https://www.goredforwomen.org/en/about-heart-disease-in-women/facts/heart-disease-linked-to-dementia-in-women.

259 Calle, "Severe Menopause symptoms Linked to Cognitive Impairment."

260 Alzheimer's Association, "2024 Alzheimer's Disease Facts and Figures," *Alzheimer's Dement* 20, no. 5 (2024), https://www.alz.org/media/Documents/alzheimers-facts-and-figures.pdf.

261 See, e.g.: M. Sochocka et al., "Cognitive Decline in Early and Premature Menopause," *International Journal of Molecular Sciences* 24, no. 7 (2023): 6566, DOI: 10.3390/ijms24076566; W. Hao et al., "Age at Menopause and All-Cause and Cause-Specific Dementia: A Prospective Analysis of the UK Biobank Cohort," *Human Reproduction* 38, no. 9 (2023): 1746, DOI: 10.1093/humrep/dead130; N. Calvo et al., "Associated Risk and Resilience Factors of Alzheimer's Disease in Women with Early Bilateral Oophorectomy: Data from The UK Biobank," *Journal of Alzheimer's Disease* 102, no. 1 (2024): 119, DOI: 10.3233/JAD-240646.

262 A. Haridasani Gupta, "How Menopause Changes the Brain," *The New York Times*, November 21, 2023, https://www.nytimes.com/2023/11/21/well/mind/menopause-dementia-risk-estrogen.html.

263 PhytoSERM to Prevent Menopause Associated Decline in Brain Metabolism and Cognition: ClinicalTrials.gov ID NCT05664477.

264 "Study Suggests Estrogen to Prevent Alzheimer's Warrants Renewed Research Interest," Weill Cornell Medicine Newsroom, October 23, 2023, https://news.weill.cornell.edu/news/2023/10/study-suggests-estrogen-to-prevent-alzheimer%E2%80%99s-warrants-renewed-research-interest.

265 Haridasani Gupta, "How Menopause Changes the Brain."

266 "Senior Women," Anxiety and Depression Association of America, accessed November 2, 2024, https://adaa.org/find-help-for/women/senior-women.

267 S. Alblooshi et al., "Does Menopause Elevate the Risk for Developing Depression and Anxiety? Results from a Systematic Review," *Australasian Psychiatry* 31, no. 2 (2023): 165, DOI: 10.1177/10398562231165439.

268 See, e.g.: N. Mishra et al., "Exercise Beyond Menopause: Dos and Dont's," *Journal of Mid-life Health* 2, no. 2 (2011): 51, DOI:

10.4103/0976-7800.92524; W. Li et al., "Effects of Exercise Programmes on Quality of Life in Osteoporotic and Osteopenic Postmenopausal Women: A Systematic Review and Meta-Analysis," *Clinical Rehabilitation* 23, no. 10 (2009): 888, DOI: 10.1177/0269215509339002.

269 See, e.g.: J. Starr, "You've Heard of Osteoporosis. What About Osteopenia?" Hospital for Special Surgery, October 1, 2021, https://www.hss.edu/article_what-is-osteopenia.asp; Haelim Lee et al., "Effects of 8-Week Pilates Exercise Program on Menopause Symptoms and Lumbar Strength and Flexibility in Postmenopausal Women," *Journal of Exercise Rehabilitation* 12, no. 3 (2016): 247, DOI: 10.12965/jer.1632630.315.

270 D. Oliveira et al., "Effect of Massage in Postmenopausal Women with Insomnia—a Pilot Study," *Clinics* 66, no. 2 (2011): 343, DOI: 10.1590/S1807-59322011000200026.

271 S. McCurry et al., "Telephone-Based Cognitive Behavioral Therapy for Insomnia in Perimenopausal and Postmenopausal Women with Vasomotor Symptoms," *The Journal of the American Medical Association Internal Medicine* 176, no. 7 (2016): 913, DOI: 10.1001/jamainternmed.2016.1795.

272 L. Hammit, "Women's Sexual Activity in Later Years Influenced by Partner Issues, UCSF Study Shows, UC San Francisco, June 24, 2009, https://www.ucsf.edu/news/2009/06/96755/womens-sexual-activity-later-years-influenced-partner-issues-ucsf-study-shows; D. Morgan and P. Malani, "Poll Shows Impact of Menopause and Other Health Issues on Older Women's Sex Lives," University of Michigan Institute for Healthcare Policy & Innovation, May 12, 2022, https://ihpi.umich.edu/news/poll-shows-impact-menopause-and-other-health-issues-older-womens-sex-lives.

273 See also: Peacock, *Menopause*.

274 Faubion et al., "The 2022 Hormone Therapy Position Statement."

275 See, e.g.: M. Nerattini et al., "Systematic Review and Meta-Analysis of the Effects of Menopause Hormone Therapy on Risk of Alzheimer's Disease and Dementia," *Frontiers in Aging Neuroscience*, no. 15 (2023), DOI: 10.3389/fnagi.2023.1260427; Calle, "Severe Menopause Symptoms Linked to Cognitive Impairment"; A. Shumaker et al., "Estrogen Plus Progestin and the Incidence of Dementia and Mild Cognitive Impairment in Postmenopausal Women," *The Journal of the American Medical Association* 289, no. 20 (2003): 2651, DOI: 10.1001/jama.289.20.2651; N. Pourhadi et al., "Menopausal Hormone Therapy

and Dementia: Nationwide, Nested Case-Control Study," *BMJ*, June 28, 2023, DOI: 10.1136/bmj-2022-072770; C. Oliver-Williams et al., "The Route of Administration, Timing, Duration and Dose of Postmenopausal Hormone Therapy and Cardiovascular Outcomes in Women: A Systematic Review," *Human Reproduction Update* 25, no. 2 (2018): 257, DOI: 10.1093/humupd/dmy039; Levin et al., "Estrogen Therapy for Osteoporosis in the Modern Era"; A. Gosset et al., "Menopausal Hormone Therapy for the Management of Osteoporosis," *Best Practice & Research Clinical Endocrinology & Metabolism* 35, no. 6 (2021): 101551, DOI: 10.1016/j.beem.2021.101551.

276 Faubion et al., "The 2022 Hormone Therapy Position Statement."

277 N. Calv et al., "Associated Risk and Resilience Factors of Alzheimer's Disease in Women with Early Bilateral Oophorectomy: Data from the UK Biobank," *Journal of Alzheimer's Disease* 102, no. 1 (2024): 119, DOI: 10.3233/JAD-240646.

278 Hurtado et al., "Weight Loss Response to Semaglutide in Postmenopausal Women."

279 A. Mahajan and R. Patni, "Menopause and Osteoarthritis: Any Association?," *Journal of Mid-life Health* 9, no. 4 (2018): 171, DOI: 10.4103/jmh.JMH_157_18; Kozinoga, "Low Back Pain in Women."

Chapter 15

280 Faubion et al., "The 2022 Hormone Therapy Position Statement."

281 Huang, "Anxiety Disorder in Menopausal Women and the Intervention Efficacy of Mindfulness-Based Stress Reduction."

282 H. Xu et al., "Effects of Mind-Body Exercise on Perimenopausal and Postmenopausal Women: A Systematic Review and Meta-Analysis," *Menopause* 31, no. 5 (2024): 457, DOI: 10.1097/GME.0000000000002336.

283 A. Haridasani Gupta and Dana G. Smith, "Is Delaying Menopause the Key to Longevity?" *The New York Times*, June 24, 2024, https://www.nytimes.com/2024/06/24/well/live/menopause-ovaries-womens-health-longevity.html.

284 See, e.g.: B. Tariq et al., "Women's Knowledge and Attitudes to the Menopause: A Comparison of Women over 40 Who Were in the Perimenopause, Post Menopause and Those Not in the Peri or Post Menopause," *BMC Women's Health* 23, no. 1 (2023): 460, DOI: 10.1186

/s12905-023-02424-x; L. Brown et al., "Investigating How Menopausal Factors and Self-Compassion Shape Well-Being: An Exploratory Path Analysis," *Maturitas* 81, no. 2 (2015): 293, DOI: 10.1016/j.maturitas.2015.03.001.

285   See, e.g.: B. Ayers et al., "The Impact of Attitudes Towards the Menopause on Women's Symptom Experience: A Systematic Review," *Maturitas* 65, no. 1 (2010): 28, DOI: 10.1016/j.maturitas.2009.

286   Lydia Brown et al., "It's Not as Bad as You Think: Menopausal Representations are More Positive in Postmenopausal Women," *Journal of Psychosomatic Obstetrics & Gynecology* 39, no. 4 (2017): 281, DOI: 10.1080/0167482X.2017.1368486.

ACKNOWLEDGMENTS

This book wouldn't be possible without the brilliance and generosity of the women whose expertise enlightened us all: Anne Fulenwider, Antoinette Hemphill, Alicia Robbins, Arielle Bayer, Adrienne Mandelberger, Alexis Cirel, Alexis Melnick, Alison Schram, Anais Hausvater, Anita Mirchandani, Ashley Austin, Beth Silverstein, Brenda Green, Brittany Barreto, Brittany Weiner, Carli Blau, Caroline Messer, Cheryl Brause, Courtney Mamuscia, Deborah Duke, Fiona Jalinoos, Jackie Giannelli, Jannine Versi, Jo Piazza, Kara Alaimo, Kara Cruz, Kathy Casey, Kyle Koeppel Mann, Leah Ansell, Lilli Dash Zimmerman, Lisa Schoenholt, Margo Lederhandler, Marra Ackerman, Melissa Ferrara, Mollie Eastman, Natalie Givargidze, Nishi Bhopal, Pooja Rajput, Randi Zinn, Rebbecca Hertel, Robyn Grosshandler, Sara Reardon, Sarah Shealy, Shieva

Ghofrany, Stephanie Falk, Susan Frankel, Taraneh Nazem, Tracy Lockwood Beckerman, and Veronica Eyo. I am so grateful to have such incredible resources in my network and my life. You are stars!

And thank you to the inspirational leaders of the current menopause movement, including but certainly not limited to Heather Hirsch, Lauren Streicher, Laura Okafor, Tamsen Fadal, and Jo LaMarca Mathisen.

This book was a dream put into print because of Claire Sielaff and the team at Ulysses Press; thank you, thank you, thank you.

Thank you to Eve Rodsky and Lauren Smith Brody for so often (and so eloquently) saying what I am thinking; you've shown me we can make a real difference for women with our words. Thank you to the amazing women who have encouraged my writing, especially my writing of this book, including Cristiana Caruso, Eve Attermann, Fran Hauser, Ingrid Zapata Read, Jennifer Marino Thibodaux, Michelle Banks, Michelle Sanford, Ruthie Friedlander, Susan Freeman, and Tatia Gordon-Troy. Thank you to Becca Kaplan, Hilary Teeman, Rachel Liebman, and Issaka Jarrah—I love being a part of weekly meetings with two therapists, two editorial experts, and a coach who always encourages positive self-talk!

Thank you to everyone I've had the pleasure of collaborating with at Keep Company, Phoebe, The Fair Play Policy Institute, and WRK/360 for all you are doing to change the world for women and caregivers. Thank you to all my other colleagues in women's empowerment and mental health who have always cheered me on, including Ariana Cohen, Dara Astmann, Dominique Pagano, Elizabeth

Baron, Elyse Kupperman, Emma Levine, Ilana Rosenberg, Jaime Gleicher, Jillian Singer, Laura Bermudez, Lindsay Liben, Lucinda Gibbons, and Tara Silber Seligson. Thank you to my EB5ever crew for keeping me laughing and supporting every career pivot. Thank you to all my friends at and through UJA; being involved has been so meaningful for me in so many ways.

I am incredibly fortunate to have friends of all ages willing to share their wisdom, including Vicki Rother, Karen Cohen, Wendy Mechanic, and Maura Carlin. I am overwhelmed with gratitude for all my girlfriends, who have supported me since my original "Do you know anything about perimenopause?" question. You've contributed your questions, your experiences, your connections, and your eagerness to read early versions. (I especially appreciate your resources, Danielle Gorelick Shlosh, your hype-woman energy, Courtney Engel, and your encouragement, Emily Mervis!) Whether I've known you for five years or 40, you've shown up for me. I love that we can be silly at any pink occasion I host, including a professional event, child's (or dog's) birthday party, or Barbie-themed karaoke celebration of midlife. I love that there is no doubt we are in this together.

Thank you to my mom, Roxana Sobie Tetenbaum, who taught me to always advocate for myself and others (with a smile). Thank you to my dad, Bob Tetenbaum, who has given me many gifts, perhaps the most valuable of which was growing up with a kind, feminist father. Thank you to my siblings, Adam Tetenbaum and Michele Tetenbaum Goodman, for your lifelong friendship and love. Thank you to my in-laws, Michelle Dorman Levin, Alan Dorman, and Karen Dorman (aka Professor MIL) for your support and contributions of trademark legal skills, pet childcare, and biology expertise. Thank you to my very smart (and very patient) bonus brothers: Jon Levin, Lowell Caulder, and Brandon Goodman.

The family I've built is the greatest joy of my life. I love you endlessly. Thank you to our pup, Tessa, who came into our lives—and got her period—at exactly the right time. Thank you to Luke and Eva, my kids and best friends, who have been proud of this project from the start and who are always willing to give me extra hugs and kisses when I'm in my office writing. Thank you to my husband, David, whose first words in response to the opportunity to write this book were: "I've been waiting for this for you. Let's do it." Thank you for the extra bedtime duties, unconditional love, and true partnership.

And thank you to you, the reader. We did it! (IYKYK.) And we're just getting started. The rest is still unwritten.

ABOUT THE AUTHOR

Lauren A. Tetenbaum, LCSW, JD, PMH-C, is a social worker specializing in supporting women through life transitions. Through her counseling practice, Lauren provides therapy to women and couples in New York, New Jersey, Connecticut, and Florida. She also facilitates groups and workshops to empower women in corporate settings and trains other mental health professionals on issues impacting women's wellness.

A former lawyer, Lauren regularly contributes thought leadership on women's rights through speaking engagements, writing, and digital media. Her areas of expertise include perinatal mental health, gender equity, working parenthood, and reproductive healthcare.

Lauren received her BA (magna cum laude) from the University of Pennsylvania before returning to her hometown of New York City to earn her MSW from New York University and JD from the Cardozo School of Law. Lauren currently lives with her husband, two children, and Cavapoo in Westchester, New York, where she is actively involved in her community.

Please connect with Lauren on Instagram (@thecounselaur) or learn more at TheCounseLaur.com.

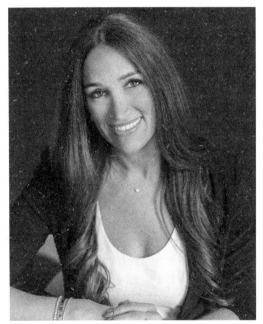

© Amanda Berce